THE ROLE OF DIGITAL HEALTH POLICY AND LEADERSHIP

Studies in Health Technology and Informatics

Internationally, health informatics is driven by developments in biomedical technologies and medical informatics research that are advancing in parallel and form one integrated world of information and communication media and result in massive amounts of health data. These components include genomics and precision medicine, machine learning, translational informatics, intelligent systems for clinicians and patients, mobile health applications, data-driven telecommunication and rehabilitative technology, sensors, intelligent home technology, EHR and patient-controlled data, and Internet of Things.

The series Studies in Health Technology and Informatics (HTI) was started in 1990 in collaboration with EU programmes that preceded the Horizon 2020 to promote biomedical and health informatics research. It has developed into a highly visible global platform for the dissemination of original research in this field, containing more than 250 volumes of high-quality works from all over the world.

The international Editorial Board selects publications with relevance and quality for the field. All contributions to the volumes in the series are peer reviewed.

Volumes in the HTI series are submitted for indexing by MEDLINE/PubMed; Web of Science: Conference Proceedings Citation Index – Science (CPCI-S) and Book Citation Index – Science (BKCI-S); Google Scholar; Scopus; EMCare.

Volume 312

Recently published in this series

ISSN 0926-9630 (print)
ISSN 1879-8365 (online)

The Role of Digital Health Policy and Leadership

From Reactive to Proactive

Edited by

Karim Keshavjee

Institute of Health Policy, Management and Evaluation,
Dalla Lana School of Public Health, University of Toronto, Canada

and

Alireza Khatami

Institute of Health Policy, Management and Evaluation,
Dalla Lana School of Public Health, University of Toronto, Canada

IOS Press

Amsterdam • Berlin • Washington, DC

ISBN 978-1-64368-494-9 (print)
ISBN 978-1-64368-495-6 (online)
Library of Congress Control Number: 2024931118
doi: 10.3233/SHTI312

Cover illustration © Zohar Shachak. Reproduced with permission.

Publisher
IOS Press BV
Nieuwe Hemweg 6B
1013 BG Amsterdam
Netherlands
e-mail: order@iospress.nl

For book sales in the USA and Canada:
IOS Press, Inc.
6751 Tepper Drive
Clifton, VA 20124
USA
Tel.: +1 703 830 6300
Fax: +1 703 830 2300
sales@iospress.com

Preface

Many healthcare-system interest holders in Canada lightheartedly debate whether the Canadian Healthcare System is truly a 'system'? Several have called it the 'non-system'. We will settle the debate for good right now. The way our healthcare is organized is indeed a system, it is, however, a flawed one. The fact that feedback loops are poorly structured, that critical information is not available or accessible, and that important elements of a system are not in place is attributable to those who are the stewards and governors of the system, and not the fault of the system itself. We get what we design.

Arguably, the Canadian healthcare system is more reactive than proactive. In other words, our priorities as a system are to spend our limited resources on treating illness rather than on preventing the occurrence of diseases. We pour resources into shortening waiting lists and purchasing the latest productivity-enhancing technologies in the glorious hope that soon, very soon, we will turn the corner and finally get ahead of all the surgeries and procedures that need to be done, and everyone in Canada will be healthy again. We try to reassure ourselves that this is not a vain hope, but in our heart of hearts we know that perhaps we need to take another route.

The Future of Health Leadership, Informatics and Policy conference was inaugurated at the Dalla Lana School of Public Health and the Institute for Health Policy, Management and Evaluation at the University of Toronto as an initiative to bring back hope to our healthcare system. We are pleased to be working with the health informatics community at the University of Victora, the University of Waterloo, and Dalhousie University in bringing these proceedings to life.

It is our collective belief that informatics thinking and digital health technologies can change the trajectory of our current system and help to convert it to one that is more proactive. New, advanced, predictive technologies have become available which make this more possible than ever before, nevertheless, it is unlikely to occur without improved policies, regulations, and governance of our health system.

We are delighted to present the papers in this collection on the topic of From Reactive to Proactive: The Role of Digital Health Policy. It is our belief that health informatics and digital health have much to say about how our healthcare system can function more efficiently. To provide policymakers, decision makers and other stakeholders with the information they need to make better allocative decisions and intervene more effectively, informatics needs to play at the macro level, not just at the user level or the inter-organizational level.

The authors have thought deeply about the key issues that plague our healthcare system, and here they present their ideas about how to address them. The topics in this collection range from interoperability to governance, regulation of electronic medical records to addressing the needs of vulnerable populations. Some authors have discussed the roles of innovative approaches and new digital technologies – including artificial intelligence – to solve healthcare-system issues.

We hope you enjoy reading these papers and considering the creative ideas the authors have developed to solve important issues in our healthcare system to help us move From Reactive, to Proactive.

Karim Keshavjee
Assistant Professor, Teaching Stream
Program Director, Health Informatics Program
Institute for Health Policy, Management and Evaluation
Dalla Lana School of Public Health
University of Toronto

Alireza Khatami
Institute for Health Policy, Management and Evaluation
Dalla Lana School of Public Health
University of Toronto

About the Conference

Conference Name

Future of Health Leadership, Informatics and Policy (FHLIP)
Date: 22 February 2024
Venue: University of Toronto – Hart House, Great Hall

Chair

Mark Rochon, B.Commerce, MHSc
Institute of Health Management, Policy and Evaluation
Dalla Lana School of Public Health, University of Toronto

Peer-Reviewers

Raza Abidi, Dalhousie University
Elizabeth Borycki, School of Information Science, Victoria University
Jasmine Candeliere, Institute of Health Management, Policy and Evaluation (IHPME), University of Toronto
Helen Chen, University of Waterloo
Angela Copeland, Ontario Government
Shez Daya, Canadian Institute for Health Information
Helen Edwards, IHPME, University of Toronto
Karim Keshavjee, IHPME, University of Toronto
Alireza Khatami, IHPME, University of Toronto
Ben King, Santis Health
Audrey Laporte, IHPME, University of Toronto
Simon Ling, OntarioMD
Wendy Nelson, IHPME, University of Toronto
Mark Rochon, IHPME, University of Toronto
Emili Seto, IHPME, University of Toronto
Aviv Shachak, IHPME, University of Toronto
Zahra Shakeri Hossein Abad, IHPME, University of Toronto
Adil Shamji, Legislative Assembly of Ontario
Gillian Strudwick, Centre for Addiction and Mental Health
Christopher Sulway, OntarioMD
Jen Tin, Canadian Agency for Drugs and Technologies in Health
Abbas Zavar, OntarioMD

Sponsors

Dalla Lana School of Public Health, University of Toronto
Institute of Health Policy, Management and Evaluation, University of Toronto

Peer-Review Process

The call for papers was first announced on the conference webpage on 15 June 2023. The deadline for manuscript submissions was originally set as 22 September 2023, but was extended to 1 October 2023. By the deadline, 26 manuscripts had been submitted to the conference. Peer-reviewers were chosen from an expert panel of academic and non-academic health informaticians and key stakeholders in the digital health sector from across Canada. Each submission was reviewed by at least two referees. Twenty manuscripts were accepted conditionally for presentation at the conference and for publication in the conference proceedings. The decisions were sent to the authors on 30 October 2023, and they were requested to submit their revised versions no later than 14 November 2023. One author then withdrew their paper. Final decision letters were sent to the authors on 15 December 2023, and at the end of the peer-review process, 19 papers were accepted for presentation and publication.

Contents

Health Informatics Research and Innovation

Patient-Focused Technologies

Digital Transformation of the Healthcare System

The Role of Digital Health Policy and Leadership
K. Keshavjee and A. Khatami (Eds.)

doi:10.3233/SHTI231301

A Framework for Implementing Disease Prevention and Behavior Change Evidence at Scale

Karim KESHAVJEE[a,1], Jasmine CANDELIERE[a], Felipe CEPEDA[a], Manmohan MITTAL[a], Shawar ALI[a] and Aziz GUERGACHI[a,b,c]

[a] *Institute of Health, Policy and Management, Dalla Lana School of Public Health, University of Toronto, Toronto, ON, Canada*
[b] *Department of Information Technology Management, Ted Rogers School of Management, Toronto Metropolitan University, Toronto, ON, Canada*
[c] *Department of Mathematics and Statistics, York University, Toronto, ON, Canada*
ORCiD ID: Karim Keshavjee https://orcid.org/0000-0003-1317-7035

Abstract. The current corpus of evidence-based information for chronic disease prevention and treatment is vast and growing rapidly. Behavior change theories are increasingly more powerful but difficult to operationalize in the current healthcare system. Millions of Canadians are unable to access personalized preventive and behavior change care because our in-person model of care is running at full capacity and is not set up for mass education and behavior change programs. We propose a framework to utilize data from electronic medical records to identify patients at risk of developing chronic disease and reach out to them using digital health tools that are overseen by the primary care team. The framework leverages emerging technologies such as artificial intelligence, digital health tools, and patient-generated data to deliver evidence-based knowledge and behavior change to patients across Canada at scale. The framework is flexible to enable new technologies to be added without overwhelming providers, patients or implementers.

Keywords. population diabetes prevention, risk profiling, behavior change theory, patient segmentation, digital health.

1. Introduction

Primary care in Canada is overwhelmed. A primary care physician with a typical 2000-patient roster needs to spend 13 hours *per day* to provide all the evidence-based preventive and chronic disease management interventions available today [1]. The current corpus of medical knowledge doubles every 73 days, which will only increase that workload over time [2]. The primary care, in-person model of care, is simply incapable of delivering the necessary preventive and prophylactic care already available. We need a new paradigm to make our healthcare system more proactive.

We use diabetes prevention as a case study to design a different approach to patient engagement and intervention. Over 5.7 million Canadians are at risk of developing

---

[1] Corresponding Author: Karim Keshavjee, karim.keshavjee@utoronto.ca

diabetes over the next decade, yet diabetes is largely preventable with simple, proven interventions. Our research question was inspired by the Centers for Disease Control and Prevention's (CDC's) behavioral economics model of population-level diabetes prevention [3]. Namely, "What is the evidence base for large-scale delivery of prevention and behavior change directly to consumers at the lowest possible cost?"

2.   Method

We combined the AIDA (Awareness, Interest, Desire, and Action) marketing framework [4], the Transtheoretical Model of behavior change (TTM) (Pre-contemplation, Contemplation, Determination, Action, Relapse, Maintenance) [5], and Self-determination Theory (SDT) [6] to develop the core of our patient engagement framework. We decided to use a direct marketing approach instead of the community advertising and organic awareness approach used by the CDC [3] since we expect to work with health service organizations that already have a database of patients in their electronic medical record systems, laboratory information systems, or pharmacy management systems. Utilizing a variety of healthcare services will allow us to capture a wider range of I@Rs, given that many people may not have a primary care physician or attend appointments regularly. Direct marketing is also much more targeted and therefore less costly than advertising and promotion. The framework was revised and validated through extensive stakeholder consultation (N>50), including patient representatives, healthcare providers, policymakers, researchers, and behavioral experts. Our research team is named PREVENT (PRoactive Ecosystem for Values, Exercise, Nutrition and Therapeutics). Ethics approval was not obtained for this co-design project.

3.   Results

3.1. The patient journey for large-scale disease prevention and treatment

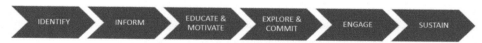

Figure 1. The PREVENT patient journey.

We identified 6 stages in our direct-to-patient journey model, as illustrated in Figure 1. 1) IDENTIFY utilizes risk profiling tools (e.g., risk scores and predictive AI and ML) to identify individuals at highest risk (I@R) of developing a disease. 2) INFORM is a systematic approach for reaching out to those at risk through patient portals, letters, and phone calls on behalf of a trusted healthcare provider or provider that the patient has previously interacted with. I@R are asked to download a digital health application (app) which will 3) EDUCATE and MOTIVATE them using a variety of evidence-based behavior change theories (satisfies part of the Mastery component of self-determination theory (SDT)) [6]. I@R who do not respond to portal messages or letters are referred to a health coach contracted to the clinic who will reach out by phone to the individual directly. When the I@R is sufficiently educated and motivated, they are invited to 4) EXPLORE their options and to set a goal for, or, to COMMIT to one option (satisfies the Autonomy and part of the Mastery components of SDT). During the Explore stage, I@R are offered either a peer-to-peer group intervention or a health coach [7]. 5) In the ENGAGE stage, I@R interact with their coach or their peers (satisfies the Relationship component of SDT) to work on the goal they selected in the Commit stage. 6) The SUSTAIN stage provides I@R the motivation, support, habits, and structure to continue on their journey of health.

3.2. What needs to be true?

We identified the key components of a digital infrastructure required to deliver the interventions contemplated by the model, at scale. These include, 1) a data extraction and risk profiling infrastructure that can extract data from electronic medical record systems and generate lists of patients at risk of developing various chronic diseases. 2) Psychographic and demographic segmentation of I@R to ensure communications are tailored to the individual's worldview and language and that they are maximally attracted to the program. 3) Apps that can be easily skinned to the patient's preferences based on their demographics (younger/older, male/female, language, etc.) to provide demographic customization to the app. 4) Apps that educate at the level of the individual's health literacy, utilize established behavior change techniques, and are responsive to the changing needs of users. 5) Ability to package existing real-world interventions (health coaches, weight loss programs, gyms, nutritionists, etc.) into a tailored package for the I@R based on preferences and resource availability (e.g., insurance coverage, time, etc). 6) Ability to provide components of multiple behavior change theories consistently in the entire experience. 7) Assist I@R in developing healthy habits instead of behavior change. There is a small, but increasing literature demonstrating that habit formation, i.e., repeating the same behavior in the same context until it becomes automatic and effortless, may take longer to acquire but requires less ongoing effort to sustain [8]. 8) An experimentation framework that allows testing of potential interventions for efficacy and effectiveness for different segments/populations of patients.

3.3. Leveraging AI in achieving platform goals

Artificial intelligence (AI) and machine learning can analyze health records, lifestyle choices, and genetic predispositions to identify individuals at high risk using predictive analytics. Using novel prescriptive analytics [9], AI can also help develop personalized interventions rooted in medical data, individual psychological tendencies, and a deep understanding of clinical practice guidelines

The melding of AI with behavioral economic concepts, such as loss aversion, refines this profiling, allowing interventions tailored to health risks and psychological readiness. AI's ability to monitor real-time feedback, glean insights from behavior data, and recommend tailored actions during the ENGAGE stage, can help ensure personalized and impactful engagement. This synergy, combining AI's capabilities with insights from behavioral economics and behavior change theories, could lead to a transformative healthcare landscape.

3.4. Policy options for disease prevention at scale

There are several policy options available for disease prevention at scale. Option 1 (Primary Care), the current approach, is to expect that primary care physicians or their teams will do this type of work. This approach has not worked in the 2 decades since diabetes prevention programs have become well-described and proven [10], and we argue that, given the shortage of family physicians and the huge amount of time required to address this population-level issue, it is unlikely to work over the next 2 decades.

Option 2 (Telehealth) is to provide specialized telehealth programs for population health management as they have done in the US [11]. This approach has been shown to be effective but has not been scalable to date. Referral rates, which depend on physicians detecting the disease opportunistically, are low. Telehealth programs are cost-effective, but it is difficult to imagine that a telehealth prevention program could scale up to serving close to 6 million individuals at risk of developing diabetes.

Option 3 (Digital Health) has the benefit of using data that already exists to prospectively identify patients at the highest risk. Targeting high-risk individuals has been shown to reduce utilization of the healthcare system, and thus has a favorable return on investment. Using marketing approaches means leveraging consumer engagement platforms, a relatively mature technology, for population health management. Consumers appreciate the marketing approach and patients are likely to appreciate it too. It would certainly enable healthcare to finally provide services in a manner that consumers are used to getting in other industries. Consumer engagement platforms provide many of the functions listed in the What needs to be true section. The peer-to-peer format is particularly compelling, as it promises to lower costs and not require scarce and overworked clinicians to get involved in chronic disease prevention.

3.5. Recommendations for new policies

We recommend that governments and other stakeholders interested in delivering high-quality and high-fidelity proven interventions to large numbers of individuals, invest in key components of the infrastructure proposed above which will be needed regardless of which model of care moves forward or whether multiple models are implemented. For example, the data extraction and patient identification platform will be necessary for ensuring the population-level reach of any future intervention. Invest in an experimentation platform so that mobile apps and other interventions can be tested quickly to generate appropriate evidence for population-based dissemination.

4.   Discussion

The pressing need for a proactive paradigm in healthcare, highlighted by the intensifying demands on primary care in Canada, requires innovative approaches. The methodology presented utilizes patient-specific data, evidence-based information on patient care, the principles of behavioral economics, behavior change theory, habit development and artificial intelligence to create population-level interventions that work at scale and are individually and economically sustainable.

This model stands out for its nuanced acknowledgment of the diverse nature of healthcare consumers. It signifies an evolutionary step in preventive healthcare by emphasizing psychographic segmentation and tailoring applications based on a mix of demographic and health literacy parameters. Furthermore, the move from behavioral change to the establishment of enduring habits in a peer-to-peer setting offers a sustainable solution to a complex problem.

There are several limitations to the model proposed which need further research. 1. Assumption of rationality: behavioral theories often rely on rational actors. However, in real-world healthcare, emotions, misinformation, deep-rooted beliefs and varying cultural norms can cause deviations from expected behavior. 2. Infrastructure: Setting up the proposed digital infrastructure is likely to be challenging, requiring the cooperation of several stakeholders in the healthcare system, including physicians, vendors and government. Communicating the concept to citizens so that they understand the benefits of the platform will also be challenging. 3. Engagement risks: The assumption that healthcare consumers universally appreciate a marketing approach may be overly optimistic. Health communications may be received differently than conventional marketing content. Ensuring that physicians participate in the platform and encourage patient participation will be key to the success of such a project. 4. Ethical implications: A broader application of this model could raise concerns over the ethical use of patient data, especially with strategic intervention targeting. Good governance and ethical oversight will be an important adjunct to ensuring the success of the project.

5. Conclusion

The PREVENT initiative is exploring a variety of futuristic architectures that enable outreach to millions of patients with high fidelity to proven interventions while leveraging existing institutions and infrastructure. This paper presents one potential architecture for disease prevention for I@R of developing chronic diseases.

References

[1]   Porter J, Boyd, C, Skandari MR, Laiteerapong N. Revisiting the Time Needed to Provide Adult Primary Care. J Gen Intern Med. 2023; 147–155. https://doi.org/10.1007/s11606-022-07707-x

[2]   Densen P. Challenges and opportunities facing medical education. Trans Am Clin Climatol Assoc. 2011;122:48-58. PMID: 21686208; PMCID: PMC3116346.

[3]   Soler RE, Proia K, Jackson MC, Lanza A, Klein C, Leifer J, Darling M. Nudging to Change: Using Behavioral Economics Theory to Move People and Their Health Care Partners Toward Effective Type 2 Diabetes Prevention. Diabetes Spectr. 2018 Nov;31(4):310-319. doi: 10.2337/ds18-0022.

[4]   Hanlon A. The AIDA model and how to apply it in the real world. SmartInsights. 2023 Mar; Available at https://tinyurl.com/rcd85pkd. Accessed Sept 13, 2023.

[5]   Hashemzadeh M, Rahimi A, Zare-Farashbandi F, Alavi-Naeini AM, Daei A. Transtheoretical Model of Health Behavioral Change: A Systematic Review. Iran J Nurs Midwifery Res. 2019 Mar-Apr;24(2):83-90. doi: 10.4103/ijnmr.IJNMR_94_17.

[6]   Phillips AS, Guarnaccia CA. Self-determination theory and motivational interviewing interventions for type 2 diabetes prevention and treatment: A systematic review. J Health Psychol. 2020 Jan;25(1):44-66. doi: 10.1177/1359105317737606.

[7]   Golkhandan E, Paglialonga A, Guergachi A, Lussier MT, Richard C, Dube L, et al. Design for a Virtual Peer-to-Peer Knowledge to Action Platform for Type 2 Diabetes. Stud Health Technol Inform. 2022 May 25;294:614-618. doi: 10.3233/SHTI220542.

[8]   Ma H, Wang A, Pei R, Piao M. Effects of habit formation interventions on physical activity habit strength: meta-analysis and meta-regression. Int J Behav Nutr Phys Act. 2023 Sep 12;20(1):109. doi: 10.1186/s12966-023-01493-3.

[9] Lenatti M, Carlevaro A, Guergachi A, Keshavjee K, Mongelli M, Paglialonga A. A novel method to derive personalized minimum viable recommendations for type 2 diabetes prevention based on counterfactual explanations. PLoS One. 2022 Nov 17;17(11):e0272825. doi: 10.1371/journal.pone.0272825.

[10] Keshavjee K, Ali S, Khatami A, Guergachi A. PREVENT Research Team. Two decade of diabetes prevention efforts: A call to innovate and revitalize our approach to lifestyle change. Diabetes Res Clin Pract. 2023 Jul;201:110680. doi: 10.1016/j.diabres.2023.110680.

[11] Centers for Medicare and Medicaid. Medicare Diabetes Prevention Program Expanded Model. https://tinyurl.com/5peatxee. Accessed Sept 13, 2023.

The Role of Digital Health Policy and Leadership
K. Keshavjee and A. Khatami (Eds.)
© 2024 The Authors.
This article is published online with Open Access by IOS Press and distributed under the terms
of the Creative Commons Attribution Non-Commercial License 4.0 (CC BY-NC 4.0).
doi:10.3233/SHTI231302

Measuring and Managing Healthcare Supply and Demand in Real-Time

Karim KESHAVJEE[a,1], Jonathan MARCUS[b], Ryan DOHERTY[c], Alireza
KHATAMI[a,d], Faiza ARSLAN[a] and Aziz GUERGACHI[a,d,e]
[a] *Institute for Health Policy, Management and Evaluation, Dalla Lana School of Public Health, University of Toronto, ON, Canada*
[b] *Dr. Jonathan Marcus Medicine Professional Corp., Toronto, ON, Canada*
[c] *Empower Inc., Toronto, ON, Canada*
[d] *Department of Information Technology Management, Ted Rogers School of Management, Toronto Metropolitan University, Toronto, ON, Canada*
[e] *Department of Mathematics and Statistics, York University, Toronto, ON, Canada*
ORCiD ID: Karim Keshavjee https://orcid.org/0000-0003-1317-7035, Alireza Khatami
https://orcid.org/0000-0002-4175-5755

Abstract. Measuring the supply and demand for access to and wait-times for healthcare is key to managing healthcare services and allocating resources appropriately. Yet, few jurisdictions in distributed, socialized medicine settings have any way to do so. In this paper, we propose the requirements for a jurisdictional patient scheduling system that can measure key metrics, such as supply of and demand for regulated health care professional care, access to and wait times for care, real-time health system utilization and provide the data to compute patient journeys. The system is also capable of tracking new supply of providers and who does not have access to a primary care provider. Benefits, limitations and risks of the model are discussed.

Keywords. Patient scheduling system, healthcare supply, healthcare demand, wait times, health system utilization, patient journey, access to care.

1. Introduction

Canada's healthcare system is in crisis. The lack of metrics for very basic characteristics of the system, such as the demand for care, the supply of care, access to care and wait times for care makes it impossible to plan or allocate resources effectively [1].

We set out to design a digital solution that could not only provide the data necessary for real-time tracking of supply and demand for healthcare services but also make it more efficient for all players in the healthcare system to transact business with each other. This paper provides design and architectural specifications for a jurisdiction-level scheduling system that enables patients and providers to book appointments, while also providing system planners and managers actionable supply and demand metrics for health system management in loosely coupled health systems.

---

[1] Corresponding Author: Karim Keshavjee, karim.keshavjee@utoronto.ca

2.   Method

We identified key supply and demand metrics that are missing in the Canadian healthcare system because of the distributed and loosely coupled nature of healthcare organizations and the lack of integration between them. We conducted a literature review of jurisdictional patient scheduling systems to identify features and issues with existing jurisdictional schedulers.   We utilized Roger Martin's Playing to Win Framework and asked ourselves "What would have to be true?" to be able to collect the desired metrics. We developed workflow and dataflow diagrams to identify where in the system key metrics should be collected and then developed the design requirements and architectural principles for an IT infrastructure that can collect the desired data. We iterated the architecture and requirements until no more elements or requirements could be identified. We identified and discuss the risks and implications of our model.

3.   Design Requirements for a Centralized Jurisdictional Scheduling System

3.1. Functional and Data Requirements

Data required to deliver Centralized Scheduling System (CSS) benefits are shown in Table 1.   Most of the data is self-explanatory. Some are new functions and are described below. We introduce the idea of "accounts" to track important metadata that would otherwise not be available, such as whether a patient has a primary care provider and whether a physician is accepting new patients. When patients request an appointment, the system provides them with a time-limited session token. The session token ensures that unbooked appointments are tracked and measurable.

Emergency departments (ED) and hospitals should have their admission, discharge and transfer (ADT) systems integrated to the CSS. This ensures that the system is able to track ED and hospital utilization, just as it would be able to track primary care and specialist utilization, even though they do not typically book appointments with patients.

Common issues with jurisdictional patient scheduling systems include inability to address the heterogeneity of needs of participating organizations and making scheduling easier does not automatically increase the Provider supply [1]. Online schedulers can improve patient satisfaction with the appointment booking process and decrease no-show rates if reminders are included in the system, and if patients are provided with the choice of reminder by email or SMS [2]. The ability to book another physician in the same clinic or at a walk-in clinic or virtual care clinic, depending on urgency is also valued by patients [3].

3.2.   Metrics required to manage the healthcare system

Table 1. Metrics and Data for Monitoring the Healthcare System.

Metric	Measure	Data Needed
Supply	# MDs Accepting new patients # Appointments available aggregate # Appointments available for a patient population	Accepting new patient flag MD appointments slots, next 6 months, rolling # Patients in roster Provider specialty Provider availability preferences
Demand	# Patients needing a doctor # Location of patients needing a doctor # Forecast demand for appointments	Primary care physician FSA associated with patient location Average # visits per patient per doctor Historical # of visits per patient per doctor
Supply-Demand Mismatch	# Clinics at risk of not meeting demand # Clinics with increased unutilized supply # Aggregate demand vs Aggregate supply	# of future appointments per clinic and clinician Average # visits per patient per clinic Number of patients in a practice Locations of clinics Patient population within locations
Access	# Appointment requests Appointment type requested # Appointments booked # Appointments not fulfilled	Appointment requested Appointment type requested Urgency of appointment types Appointment booked Appointment completed
Wait times	Time from first request to primary care appointment Time from referral to specialist appointment Time from specialist appointment to procedure	Time of appointment Time of referral Time of specialist appointment Time of procedure
Utilization	# ER visits # Hospitalizations # Bookings	Admitted to ER Admitted to hospital Referral to community Follow-up booking
Unfulfilled demand	Time patient has waited for a new family doctor Patient booked family doctor appointment and then went to ER, walk-in clinic, urgent care clinic, or virtual care clinic	Appointments requested – booked ER, walk-in clinic, urgent care clinic, virtual care clinic visit
Wasted Supply	% no-show rate #unfilled appointment slots	Appointment no-show Unfilled appointment slots

3.3. Non-Functional Features of the Centralized Scheduling System

The CSS enables all Users (patients, providers and healthcare facilities) to register quickly and easily with a single sign-on. The CSS should utilize existing jurisdictional Client and Provider registries to pre-populate the users of the system; the vast majority of Users should not need to create a new account; they should claim an existing account. The CSS would allow all Users to access features associated with allowed clinics based on permissions with the same account without needing to register more than once or fill out duplicative forms. The CSS provides standard scheduling services that are described below. Patients can access the scheduling services through the web, mobile apps, chatbots, voice services, or permitted third party applications. Patients can call their family doctor's office to book an appointment. If the phone line is busy, the patient's call can be automatically routed to the CSS where voice technologies enable convenient access to the standard scheduling services for all patients, regardless of Internet access. A live help desk should be available for those not comfortable with technology or who need individual assistance, which also provides the same standard set of scheduling services. The system could ask patients routine questions to calculate the time required to provide appropriate care and timeliness of appointments. A moderation function would allow clinics to manage exceptions to rules; e.g., physical examinations, therapy sessions or patients that need additional time.

3.4. User accounts and claiming a user account

User accounts can be claimed by authenticated users. Since regulated healthcare providers and local registration authorities at healthcare organizations (Providers) are the best authenticated players in the system, they should be invited to claim their accounts first. Providers would then sponsor or nominate individuals within their organization to claim their accounts. Sponsored individuals can then reach out to patients to offer them an opportunity to claim their accounts. This cascading outreach can be done through the patient portal or through other communication channels that the clinic uses. Unattached patients can be informed about their options through the 811 service or at Walk-in clinics. The cascading approach allows efficient and safe reach to the vast majority of citizens.

User accounts for the Patient role can also specify the circle of care –the healthcare providers that the patient has interacted with in the past, preferences related to healthcare providers they would like to interact with in the future (i.e. language spoken or near specific locations), and the ones that they can access directly without the need for a referral, or process for geolocation.

3.5. Provider Usage of the System

Providers can integrate their clinic schedulers with the CSS by adding an API key or API-integration credentials for their existing scheduler. All providers, meaning any and all regulated healthcare professionals, should be registered to the CSS. The integration enables 2-way synchronization of appointments. Providers can update information about their clinic location(s), hours of operation, availability for appointments, whether they are accepting new patients, and a variety of other information directly into their "account" and practice profile(s). Specialists can also include information about their specialty and subspecialties and what types of patients they do and do not see. While the CSS would have some generic rules about how appointments can be booked (e.g., patients cannot book a specialist directly, patient cannot book a doctor they have never seen before, etc.), Providers would have the ability to apply their own rules, such as "if appointment type = Physical Examination, book only after confirmation by clinic". Patients can book an appointment with a specialist if they receive a "referral token" from their family physician or the patient's account is automatically given access based on permissions associated with their health card or EMR record ID. Physicians who prefer to book their own appointments can still use the when-busy rollover to the system and synchronize their scheduler with the CSS. The system should incentivize providers to keep their availability as accurate as possible and should have at least 3 months of availability documented and/or information about how patients can access care after-hours or outside of their own availability, since patients stop using the system if they do not see appointments available in the system.

3.6. Patient Usage of the System

Patients register themselves to the system so they can book appointments. Patients update their own information on the system, including their address, and create a link to their primary care provider's account, if they have a provider; if not, they can indicate they do not have a provider. The CSS sends and rescinds appointments directly to the patient's email address, mobile phone via SMS, and usual calendar. In this system, patients can book themselves into specialist offices using the same set of standard scheduling services once they get a referral from their physician. This is enabled using a time-limited token provided to the patients to book their own appointments. Patients have access to maps and filters to enable them to find the best specialist for their needs, constrained by the service they were referred to. Reminders are sent automatically, unless the patient opts-out.

4.   Architectural Principles for the System

We propose the following architectural principles to ensure the widest possible participation and least resistance to participation.

- No privileged access. Everyone in the system should be able to see all reports and dashboards on the main website for the CSS.
- Transparency of booking rules. Patients should have a clear understanding of the rules used to book appointments.
- Patient autonomy and agency should trump convenience for system builders.
- Automated regional aggregated reporting to reduce manual efforts at regional healthcare system planning for regional public sector institutions.
- Public ownership of the platform with private competition for connected apps.

5. Opportunities and Risks of the Proposed Design

The proposed design provides many of the benefits governments want to provide to citizens, including a digital front door and improved and convenient access to care across the entire spectrum of regulated health professionals, enabling experimentation with new models of care. The design also helps connect all major digital and data users for seamless integrated care, establishes common requirements for all users, provides better health data for better care, provides access to information with fewer sign-ons and builds on Health811 services and functionality. The design is compatible with software that already exists on the market with a few small customizations to accommodate the needs of a jurisdictional scheduling system. The CSS uses well-known and well-described software architecture patterns and can be developed using custom-off-the-shelf products. All data mentioned in Table 1 is collected in the course of transactions, through the user maintaining their account and through integration with hospital ADT systems. There is no need to collect additional data. Much of the start-up data has already been collected and just needs to be populated from existing Client and Provider registries, which is a strength of the design.

Most importantly, the CSS is designed to provide health system managers the information they need to manage the healthcare system effectively, provides citizens with convenience, autonomy and easier access to care and remove administrative effort from physician practices, a win for all stakeholders involved. The design is also open to enable competition amongst vendors to serve a variety of patient and provider segments. The patient's address could be used with deprivation indices to identify equity-deserving individuals and allocate resources accordingly. Of course, patients could enter their own social information into their accounts, if they so choose.

The system design does not allow for risk-adjusted care, as disease acuity is not captured in the system, although this might be inferred through data from hospitalization and emergency department visits. Although the CSS does not directly address the issue of becoming proactive, it does provide jurisdictions the information they need to plan more effectively and allocate resources efficiently to make the system more proactive.

6. Conclusion

Governments around the world are trying to manage the complexities of a modern healthcare system. The current information systems in place are siloed, which makes it difficult to get a sense of the big picture of supply, demand, access and wait times for routine and specialized care. In this paper we propose the design of a jurisdictional patient scheduling system that can help all key stakeholders to further their goals of system planning and management, convenience, and decreased administrative burden

References

[1]   Improving Health and Health Care Worldwide | IHI - Institute for Healthcare Improvement [Internet]. Measure and Understand Supply and Demand | IHI - Institute for Healthcare Improvement; [cited 2023 Oct 2]. Available from :
      https://www.ihi.org/resources/Pages/Changes/MeasureandUnderstandSupplyandDemand.aspx

[2]   Motulsky A, Bosson-Rieutort D, Usher S, et al. Evaluation of a national e-booking system for medical consultation in primary care in a universal health system. Health Policy. 2023 May;131:104759. doi: 10.1016/j.healthpol.2023.104759.

[3]   Paré G, Trudel MC, Forget P. Adoption, use, and impact of e-booking in private medical practices: mixed-methods evaluation of a two-year showcase project in Canada. JMIR Med Inform. 2014 Sep 24;2(2):e24. doi: 10.2196/medinform.3669.

[4]   Breton M, Marshall EG, Deslauriers V, et al. COVID-19 - an opportunity to improve access to primary care through organizational innovations? A qualitative multiple case study in Quebec and Nova Scotia (Canada). BMC Health Serv Res. 2022 Jun 8;22(1):759. doi: 10.1186/s12913-022-08140-w.

The Role of Digital Health Policy and Leadership
K. Keshavjee and A. Khatami (Eds.)
© 2024 The Authors.
This article is published online with Open Access by IOS Press and distributed under the terms
of the Creative Commons Attribution Non-Commercial License 4.0 (CC BY-NC 4.0).
doi:10.3233/SHTI231303

Towards Meaningful Engagement with Clinician Advisors: Lessons Learned Co-Creating a Digital Mental Health Tool

Charlotte PAPE[a,b*], Jessica KEMP[a,b*], Iman KASSAM[a,b*], Crystal CHAN[a],
Melissa GIOVINAZZO[a], Jori JONES[a,b], Melissa MCCORMICK[a], Tara PEARCEY[a],
Dave SUMMERS[a], Matthew TSUDA[a,b], Esther YOO-PARLAN[a] and
Gillian STRUDWICK[a,b1]

[a] Centre for Addiction and Mental Health, Toronto, Ontario, Canada
[b] University of Toronto, Toronto, Ontario, Canada

Abstract. In partnership with clinician advisors, a text-based program, BeWell, was co-created to support clinician well-being at a Canadian mental health hospital. This paper briefly describes the process of designing BeWell with clinician advisors and highlights key lessons learned in engaging clinicians as advisors in the design and development of a digital health intervention. The lessons learned can serve as best practices for health systems, organizations, and researchers to consider when engaging clinicians in the design, development, and implementation of digital health interventions.

Keywords. Participatory research, digital health, mental health, implementation science, social work, occupational therapy, allied health

1. Introduction

In July of 2022, the Centre for Addiction and Mental Health (CAMH) launched a survey to identify perceived clinician documentation burden related to the electronic health record, and rates of burnout amongst nursing and health disciplines staff. Using the mini-z instrument [1], results demonstrated that 50% of Social Workers (n=49) and 23% of Occupational Therapists (n=17) reported one or more symptoms of burnout. Given the findings of the survey, it was evident that organizational strategies and interventions were needed to respond to the level of burnout reported by these health disciplines. Upon consultation with researchers and clinical leaders at the organization, a text message-based program, *BeWell*, was selected to be adapted for use by clinicians to support overall clinician wellness. Though experiences of burnout are complex and highly individual, the *BeWell* program was intended to be one of multiple strategies to support clinicians and offer a low-intensity method to support clinician wellness.

To respond effectively to the needs of Occupational Therapists and Social Workers, an advisory group of clinicians was established in an effort to co-create the *BeWell* program. Over the course of 6-months, *BeWell* was tailored for mental health clinicians at CAMH using participatory design methods. This paper will briefly describe the

---

[1] Corresponding Author: Gillian Strudwick, gillian.strudwick@camh.ca
* These authors contributed equally and share first authorship

process of designing and developing *BeWell* with clinician advisors and will highlight key lessons learned in engaging clinicians as partners in the design, development, and implementation of a digital mental health intervention for clinicians. These lessons provide insights into best practices for engaging clinicians in the design of future digital health interventions

2. Overview of *BeWell*

BeWell is a text-based population mental health intervention, which has been implemented and evaluated in previous studies [2]. As part of an organizational strategic initiative to support clinician well-being, the *BeWell* intervention has been adapted to support clinicians at CAMH. In this context, *BeWell* aims to support Social Workers and Occupational Therapists' wellbeing by connecting them to mental health resources, psychoeducational tools, supportive motivational messaging, and professional development opportunities through a 12-week two-way text messaging program.

2.1. Design, Development, and Implementation of BeWell

A multi-phased approach, guided by the principles of participatory design [3], was used to design, develop, and implement *BeWell*. Specifically, in the first phase, an interprofessional Clinician Advisory Group (CAG) was established, consisting of a proportionate number of Occupational Therapists (n=5) and Social Workers (n=5) from a variety of clinical settings across CAMH. Each clinician volunteered to participate in the advisory group and received gift cards as compensation for their time and expertise. Once the advisory group was established, phase 2 of the project commenced. In this phase, the clinician advisors, in partnership with the research team, co-created the *BeWell* program. Bi-weekly design meetings, each one hour in length, were held with the clinician advisors between February 2023 – May 2023. In these meetings, various collaborative design activities (i.e., requirements gathering, brainstorming sessions, priority sorting activities, etc.) were facilitated to ensure the text-based program was tailored to CAMH clinicians. During this phase, the clinician advisors supported user testing of the *BeWell* program, where the program was tested for technical bugs prior to the formal launch. In the third phase, *BeWell* was implemented across CAMH for use by clinicians. The implementation process was guided by a communications and implementation plan, created in partnership with the clinician advisors.

    BeWell was launched on May 1, 2023, and will be available for use by CAMH clinicians until October 9, 2023. Following the conclusion of the program, an evaluation will be conducted to understand the user's experience and satisfaction with the text-based program.

3. Lessons Learned Co-Creating *BeWell*

To understand the lessons learned in co-creating *BeWell* with the CAG better, two questions were posed to the clinician advisors; the first relating to what they believed went well with their involvement in the group and the second concerning what could have been improved with the co-creation process. Through consultations with the advisory group, a number of themes and key lessons learned were identified and are described below.

With regards to what went well with the co-creation process, the following themes were commonly described by the clinician advisors:

3.1. Fostering Meaningful Engagement and Active Collaboration

An important aspect of maintaining interest and retention within the CAG was prioritizing meaningful engagement and active collaboration. The project leads did so by eliciting the opinion of the clinician advisors through multiple avenues, such as virtual meetings, document sharing, and facilitating input sharing via email. This approach allowed for various methods of communication, either through group discussions or through individual feedback. The clinician advisors felt that their feedback was heard and received in a genuine way and appreciated the direct impact their feedback had on the refinements to the *BeWell* program. Moreover, the clinician advisors expressed gratitude for being invited to participate in the co-creation of the BeWell program, as some described often feeling disconnected from research and quality improvement programs at the organization.

3.2. Leveraging Knowledge User Expertise

The expertise of the CAG was critical in the development and design of a supportive text-based intervention for clinicians. One of the main responsibilities of the CAG was to co-create the text messages shared through the *BeWell* program. To ensure the content was appropriate, relevant, and practical for mental health clinicians, the project leads focused on leveraging the knowledge and expertise of each advisor. This approach allowed the content to be tailored to specific health disciplines, thereby ensuring the text messages and the scheduling of the messages aligned with the needs of the clinicians as end-users. Overall, the knowledge shared by the CAG made it evident that the task was not to reiterate therapeutic tools that care providers are already trained in, but instead to inspire clinicians to take time for self-care.

3.3. Providing Compensation and Incentives

The importance of compensation and incentives was reiterated by the clinician advisors as a method to sustain engagement and interest in supporting the co-creation of *BeWell*. Ahead of each advisory group meeting, the advisors were compensated for their time through $25 gift cards. The advisors appreciated that their knowledge and time was recognized as being valuable by the project team. A clinician advisor also shared that they were impressed by the successful retention of the advisory group and felt that all discussions were engaging, and solution based as opposed to deficit based. As a result, the meetings were restorative, as opposed to taxing, which encouraged clinicians to continue attending group meetings.

3.4. Establishing a Diverse Interdisciplinary Team

Given that the *BeWell* program was designed specifically for clinical staff, the clinician advisors underscored the importance of the interdisciplinary nature of the advisory group. Partnering with both clinicians, who bring forth the expertise and knowledge of clinical workflows and practice, and researchers, who have expertise in specific research and design methodologies, was crucial for the design and implementation of the *BeWell* program. Moreover, the advisors recognized that amongst the clinician advisors, each brought different perspectives given their current roles or their current setting of practice. For instance, the advisory group had representation from Occupational Therapists and Social Workers in different clinical and non-clinical areas and roles including leadership, frontline clinical programs, and non-clinical programs. This approach enabled diverse input to be captured and incorporated into the design of *BeWell*.

3.5. Ensuring a Flexible Participatory Research Design & Approach

When establishing and organizing the CAG, it was crucial to consider the competing priorities and workloads of the clinicians who were volunteering their time to co-create *BeWell*. The advisors appreciated the flexibility of the advisory group meetings, specifically due to the virtual nature of the meetings, the flexible organization and structure of the meetings and the consistent frequency of the meetings.

The clinician advisors were also asked to describe what they believed could have been improved upon in the co-creation process. Common themes are described below:

3.6. Balancing Group Dynamics and Conflicting Feedback

Some clinician advisors expressed that during group meetings, some voices at the table felt louder than others did. Variation in the clinician advisors' comfort with verbalizing their viewpoints and sharing ideas during group sessions meant that not every clinician had an equal opportunity to contribute fulsome opinions during meetings. As a result, the more expressive voices likely exercised more influence over the project direction. Additionally, clinicians' perspectives occasionally conflicted, which required a careful approach to balancing incongruous group feedback. Managing project expectations, finding compromises, as well as clarifying project intentions and end-goals helped with determining which feedback to prioritize and which suggestions to implement into the design of the program.

3.7. Considering Workload and Time Constraints of Clinician Advisors

Clinician advisors voiced that having protected time outside of their regular clinical roles to engage in program development and user testing would have been valuable. Managing project responsibilities on top of demanding clinical roles placed an additional burden on already time constrained clinicians. The clinician advisors felt that only having the duration of Clinical Advisory Group meetings allocated to work on program deliverables, while beneficial, was challenging especially when there were tasks to complete outside of the designated meetings. Having a set period for project engagement would allow the advisors to be more involved throughout the project and enable them to contribute well-developed ideas.

3.8. Increasing the Frequency of Follow-Up with Clinician Advisors

The co-creation process established a bi-weekly meeting schedule to allow time to develop the *BeWell* program while minimizing additions to clinician workload. To continue collaboration between meeting intervals, project leads would engage clinician advisors by eliciting requests for feedback through multiple avenues. However, some clinician advisors shared that having more frequent opportunities to discuss project contents before confirming final outputs would be desirable. Clinician advisors suggested having further discussions about the content of *BeWell* messages prior to their inclusion in the program. Specifically, clinician advisors required additional time to conduct a more thorough and critical review of resources and message contents, to ensure an evidence-based approach was being employed.

3.9. Being Mindful of the Disconnect Between Funder Requirements and Project Cycles

Although clinician advisors noted that the overall program was well-organized and allowed for suitable time to accomplish outlined project goals, additional time to complete the project deliverables would have been an asset. Unfortunately, as was the case with *BeWell*, most research projects are constrained by tight timelines determined by external project funders. Clinicians noted that having longer project timelines would have allowed sufficient time to review and make modifications to project outputs.

4. Key Considerations for Future Digital Health Programs and Initiatives

While the lessons learned in co-creating the *BeWell* program are specific to the experiences of the clinician advisors involved, they may be applicable to future digital health programs and initiatives that rely on the expertise of clinician end-users. The insights gleaned from the experiences of the clinician advisors highlight the importance of maintaining flexibility, fostering a sense of community, balancing diverse perspectives, and sustaining open communication in an often rigid and time constrained research environment. Moreover, the learnings signal a need for future digital health initiatives to veer away from a 'one-size-fits-all' approach, especially with regards to methods of communicating and knowledge sharing. Being mindful of varying communication styles and preferences is imperative to ensure all voices are heard and considered equally.

As described in previous studies [4,5], clinicians are interested in being active participants in organizational initiatives, including that of research and quality improvement programs. However, despite interest, clinicians often face barriers in participating in such initiatives due to the demands of patient care and the lack of structural supports to initiate and contribute through protected time (i.e., engaging in non-clinical activities and access to funding). To enable further meaningful and active participation in initiatives outside the purview of clinical care, healthcare organizations should consider promoting opportunities for clinician participation in various initiatives while also implementing policies and procedures to afford them protected time.

The lessons learned from the design, development, and implementation of *BeWell* serve as findings for health systems, organizations, and researchers to consider when engaging clinicians in digital health programs and initiatives.

References

[1] Tajirian T, Stergiopoulos V, Strudwick G, Sequeira L, Sanches M, Kemp J, et al. The Influence of Electronic Health Record Use on Physician Burnout: Cross-Sectional Survey. J Med Internet Res. 2020 Jul 15;22(7):e19274.

[2] Risling T, Carlberg C, Kassam I, Moss T, Janssen P, Iduye S, Strudwick G. Supporting population mental health and wellness during the COVID-19 pandemic in Canada: protocol for a sequential mixed-method study. BMJ Open. 2021 Nov 18;11(11):e052259.

[3] Vaughn LM, Jacquez F. Participatory Research Methods – Choice Points in the Research Process. J Particip Res Methods. 2020 Jul 21 [cited 2023 Sep 14];1(1). Available: https://jprm.scholasticahq.com/article/13244-participatory-research-methods-choice-points-in-the-research-process.

[4] Wenke R, Noble C, Weir KA, Mickan S. What influences allied health clinician participation in research in the public hospital setting: a qualitative theory-informed approach. BMJ Open. 2020 Aug 20;10(8):e036183.

[5] Goldstein KM, Gierisch JM, Tucker M, Williams JW Jr, Dolor RJ, Henderson W. Options for Meaningful Engagement in Clinical Research for Busy Frontline Clinicians. J Gen Intern Med. 2021 Jul;36(7):2100–4.

Health Informatics: Policy and Leadership

The Role of Digital Health Policy and Leadership
K. Keshavjee and A. Khatami (Eds.)
© 2024 The Authors.
This article is published online with Open Access by IOS Press and distributed under the terms
of the Creative Commons Attribution Non-Commercial License 4.0 (CC BY-NC 4.0).
doi:10.3233/SHTI231305

Mental Health and Addiction Data Use Cases: Macro Perspectives in Ontario

Alexander DARE[a]

[a] *Institute of Health Policy, Management and Evaluation, University of Toronto, Dalla Lana School of Public Health, Toronto, ON, Canada*

Abstract. The opioid crisis in Ontario has led to a surge in preventable overdose deaths. Challenges in the mental health and addiction system, along with various contributing factors, have amplified this crisis. Underutilization of data exacerbates service gaps and hinders innovative solutions. Through stakeholder engagement, interrelated problems emerged, emphasizing the pervasive data underutilization. This research explores data usage in mental health and addictions, focusing on the opioid epidemic in Ontario and comparative jurisdictions. To improve service quality, Ontario should implement a comprehensive data management strategy. Two key recommendations include increased investment in exploring additional data use cases and evaluating policy initiatives using dynamic models throughout a patient's journey.

Keywords. Data usage, mental health, opioid crisis, underutilization, service gaps, data management

1. Background

In March 2020, Ontario unveiled its long-awaited strategic plan, "Roadmap to Wellness: A Plan to Build Ontario's Mental Health and Addiction System," to address the growing challenges in mental health and addiction. The plan envisions an integrated and connected ecosystem, emphasizing investments in data assets for system improvement. Ontario has proposed a $3.8 billion investment over the next decade, including targeted federal funds, to implement the strategic plan. This financial commitment aims to bridge the funding gap and position Ontario and Canada competitively in mental health and addiction spending compared to their OECD counterparts [1].

The COVID-19 pandemic placed a considerable strain on the limited healthcare resources available in recent years, as health officials struggled to contain the disease's numerous manifestations. Furthermore, the pandemic worsened the opioid overdose epidemic leading to an unprecedented increase in overdose-related mortality [2]. This report focuses on the macro health system level, exploring applications of mental health and addiction data, with a specific emphasis on addressing the opioid crisis.

2. Methods

The methodology comprised 14 stakeholder interviews spanning mental health, addiction services, and data management. Interviews explored data utilization in

Ontario's opioid crisis. Qualitative content analysis revealed themes and was validated by stakeholders. Comparative analysis with other crisis-prone regions was conducted. Ethical considerations were observed, and limitations included a small sample size and qualitative data focus.

3.   Results and Discussion

This compilation of mental health and addiction data use cases in Ontario is not exhaustive; instead, it specifically emphasizes macro-level perspectives.

3.1. Current State: Macro Level Applications of Mental Health and Addiction Data

3.1.1.   Mental Health and Addiction Data and Digital Initiatives (MHA DDI)

The mental health and addiction (MHA) data and digital initiatives align with the Ontario Ministry of Health's Digital First for Health strategy and have a prominent place in the "Roadmap to Wellness Plan". At a high level, the MHA Data and Digital Initiatives include the Provincial Data Set (PDS), Measurement-Based Care Solution for Ontario Structured Psychotherapy, MHA EHR Data Set and Data Analytics. Together, these four use cases support the goal of advancing real-time access and linking of patient and provider information across the mental health and addiction care continuum [1].

3.1.2.   Institute for Clinical Evaluative Sciences (ICES) Research and Analytics

The ICES mental health dashboard is a public reporting tool that monitors and evaluates Ontario's mental health and addiction system. Established in 2013 as part of the Ontario Mental Health System Reporting, the dashboard provides quarterly updates on trends and performance indicators. Drawing from multiple sources, such as the Discharge Abstract Database (DAD) etc., ICES dashboard offers a succinct summary of key data, influencing factors, and access to care [3].

Recent legal designation empowers ICES to receive Coroner data under PHIPA and the Coroners Act. This allows secure integration with Ontario's Narcotics Monitoring System data, enabling the analysis of opioid-overdose-related mortality and its correlation with opioid prescribing practices province-wide.

3.1.3.   Ontario Mental Health Reporting System (OMHRS)

The Ontario Mental Health Reporting System (OMHRS), overseen by the Canadian Institute for Health Information (CIHI), captures clinical, administrative, and demographic data for individuals receiving in-hospital mental health and addiction services in Ontario. This system, utilizing the Resident Assessment Instrument for Mental Health (RAI-MH), provides comprehensive insights, including mental health assessments, service usage, care planning, and case-mix funding applications [4]. Developed collaboratively by interRAI, the Ontario Ministry of Health, and the Ontario Health Association, the RAI-MH instrument covers key data sets, quality indicators, and clinical evaluation methods for in-patient psychiatry. Published quarterly, OMHRS offers a valuable snapshot of mental health and addiction services in the province [4].

3.1.4.   Public Health Ontario (PHO) Interactive Opioid Tool

The Interactive Opioid Tool, a collaboration between Public Health Ontario and the Ontario Ministry of Health, provides users with recent aggregate-level data on opioid-related mortality and morbidity in Ontario. This surveillance tool allows the display of figures for public health units based on factors such as age, gender, and Local Health Integration Network. Data sources include emergency department visits, hospitalizations, opioid-related deaths, and population estimates [5].

3.1.5.   Ontario's Narcotics Monitoring System (NMS)

The Narcotics Monitoring System (NMS) in Ontario is a centralized database for real-time reviews of controlled substance prescribing and dispensing at the point of care. Pharmacies upload data, and the NMS conducts audits, identifying issues like polypharmacy. Pharmacies receive immediate notifications for necessary actions. The system, operational since April 16, 2012, utilizes dispensing data from all pharmacies regardless of payment method. Notably, physicians are barred from patient-level data access, integrated into the province's upgraded medication management system [6].

3.1.6.   Drug and Alcohol Treatment Information System (DATIS)

The Drug and Alcohol Treatment Information System is a client-based information system that provides reports on Ontario's publicly funded addiction treatment services. It is intended that agencies involved in the delivery of healthcare for individuals with substance use disorders will upload demographic information about individuals who utilize their services. DATIS provides information regarding trends in substance use and how they are affected by treatment program enrollment. The database is useful for tracking patients throughout their healthcare journey and identifying the most effective treatment services. Approximately 180 partner organizations in Ontario use Catalyst (an electronic client management system) to pull information into DATIS [7].

3.2. Future State: Macro Level Applications of Mental Health and Addiction Data

3.2.1.   Cascade of Care Model

Comparable to the cascade of care model that was developed and proved effective for managing HIV and AIDS in 2017, stakeholders observing the pattern of the opioid crisis are requesting a similar framework to combat the opioid epidemic. In many circumstances, the need for services is detected by a system that is not equipped to provide adequate care. The result is that persons with opioid use disorder struggle to find the help they need while navigating a confusing system. Such persons frequently gravitate to emergency departments when more appropriate and efficient care options are available in community-based settings [8].

3.2.2.   System Dynamic Modeling

Researchers in Portland, Oregon, addressed the concern of non-medical opioid usage and accidental poisoning by developing a dynamic model. The model aimed to understand the behavioral factors contributing to patients abusing pharmaceutical opioids for non-medical purposes. Utilizing data from sources including the National Survey on Drug Use and Health (NSDUH), Treatment Episode Data Set (TEDS), Monitoring the Future (MTF) Public-Use Cross-Sectional Datasets, Automated Reports and Consolidated Ordering System (ARCOS), the model successfully predicted behavior patterns in patient populations prone to pharmaceutical opioid abuse [9].

3.2.3.   Integrated Data Warehouse

The Ontario Health Data Platform (OHDP) is an integrated data warehouse that is facilitating groundbreaking COVID-19 research. Similarly, developing an information management architecture that connects siloed data sources held separately to enable research on the opioid overdose epidemic has become critical. In response to the opioid crisis, Massachusetts established an integrated public health warehouse that connects patient-level administrative data from over twenty different sources. By investigating big data solutions for the opioid overdose epidemic, Massachusetts hopes to gain a better understanding of the clinically significant relationships that are fueling the opioid epidemic, as well as the added benefit of being able to model a patient's journey across the health system, among other things [10]. Figure 1 demonstrates the current state mental health and addiction data use cases in Ontario and potential future state scenarios.

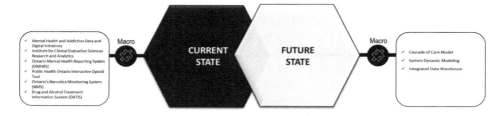

Figure 1. Visual representation of current state mental health and addiction data use cases in Ontario and potential future state scenarios.

4.   Conclusion

In practice, leveraging data is crucial for providing high-quality care and enhancing accountability within the mental health and addiction system. It is imperative to establish transparent accountability guidelines for Ontario's mental health and addiction data resources [1]. The recommendations in this study emanate from a thorough research process that integrates systematic analysis and active engagement with stakeholders. Informed by a literature review, extensive data collection, and insightful stakeholder interactions, these recommendations are designed to be both actionable and firmly grounded in empirical evidence. Specifically, the study advocates for increased resource allocation in Ontario to expand the exploration of additional data use cases at both micro and meso levels. Furthermore, it suggests that health system planners should adopt dynamic models to comprehensively assess policy initiatives throughout all stages of a patient's healthcare journey.

References

[1]　Ontario Ministry of Health. Roadmap to wellness: a plan to build Ontario's mental health and addictions system [Internet]. 2020. Available from: https://www.ontario.ca/page/roadmap-wellness-plan-build-ontarios-mental-health-and-addictions-syste m

[2]　Special Advisory Committee on the Epidemic of Opioid Overdoses. Opioid and Stimulant-related Harms in Canada. Ottawa: Public Health Agency of Canada; 2021. 71 p.

[3]　Institute for Clinical and Evaluative Sciences. Mental Health and Addictions Dashboard [Internet]. 2022. Available from: https://www.ices.on.ca/Research/Research-programs/Mental-Health-and-Addictions/MHA-Dashboard

[4]　Canadian Institute for Health Information. Ontario Mental Health Reporting System Metadata [Internet]. 2022. Available from: https://www.cihi.ca/en/ontario-mental-health-reporting-system-metadata

[5]　Public Health Ontario. Interactive Opioid Tool [Internet]. Ontario Agency for Health Protection and Promotion; 2022. Available from: https://www.publichealthontario.ca/en/data-and-analysis/substance-use/interactive-opioid-tool

[6]　Ontario Ministry of Health and Long-Term Care. Narcotics Monitoring System [Internet]. 2021. Available from: http://www.health.gov.on.ca/en/pro/programs/drugs/ons/monitoring_system.aspx

[7]　Canadian Mental Health Association. DATIS of vital importance to Ontario's addictions sector [Internet]. 2022. Available from: https://network.cmha.ca/datis-of-vital-importance-to-ontarios-addictions-sector/

[8]　Blanco C, Wiley TRA, Lloyd JJ, Lopez MF, Volkow ND. America's opioid crisis: the need for an integrated public health approach. Transl Psychiatry [Internet]. 2020;10(1):1–13. Available from: http://dx.doi.org/10.1038/s41398-020-0847-1

[9]　Wakeland W, Nielsen A, Geissert P. Dynamic model of nonmedical opioid use trajectories and potential policy interventions. Am J Drug Alcohol Abuse. 2015;41(6):508–18.

[10]　Evans EA, Delorme E, Cyr KD, Geissler KH. The Massachusetts public health data warehouse and the opioid epidemic: A qualitative study of perceived strengths and limitations for advancing research. Prev Med Reports [Internet]. 2022;28(January):101847. Available from: https://doi.org/10.1016/j.pmedr.2022.101847.

The Role of Digital Health Policy and Leadership
K. Keshavjee and A. Khatami (Eds.)
© 2024 The Authors.
This article is published online with Open Access by IOS Press and distributed under the terms
of the Creative Commons Attribution Non-Commercial License 4.0 (CC BY-NC 4.0).
doi:10.3233/SHTI231306

From Strategy to Synergy: Paving Ontario's Proactive Path in Precision Medicine with Collaboration and Visionary Leadership

Abbas ZAVAR[a][1] and Razieh POORANDY[a]

[a]Institute of Health Policy, Management and Evaluation, Dalla Lana School of Public Health, University of Toronto, Toronto, ON, Canada

ORCiD ID: Abbas Zavar https://orcid.org/0000-0003-0639-2765

Abstract. Ontario is shifting to a Precision Medicine (PM) model, which emphasizes tailored patient care, an initiative reflected in the formation of Ontario Health Teams. However, this shift faces significant data governance, policy formulation, and technology integration hurdles. To overcome these barriers, we advocate for a comprehensive PM framework to orchestrate collaboration among healthcare providers, policymakers, and technologists. This framework enhances data management, propels digital health innovations, and uphold ethical standards in AI applications. Effective deployment of this framework is crucial for actualizing PM's promise in Ontario, potentially revolutionizing healthcare delivery.

Keywords. Precision Medicine, framework, ecosystem, policymaking, digital health

1. Introduction

Ontario is at the cusp of a healthcare transformation, shifting from the traditional 'one-size-fits-all' evidence-based medicine to a more patient-centric approach. The creation of Ontario Health Teams (OHT) is a testament to this paradigm shift, aiming to improve patient outcomes through cohesive care teams [1]. Precision Medicine (PM) stands out as an ideal manifestation of this patient-centric philosophy, promising individualized care tailored to each patient's unique genetic, environmental, lifestyle and social determinants of health (SDoH) factors [2,3]. The optimal brief description for Precision Medicine is that it involves delivering the right clinical intervention—whether that be diagnosis, treatment, or prevention—at the right time, tailored specifically to the right individual [2]. PM stands as a beacon of modern medical innovation with the promise to revolutionize healthcare outcomes by ensuring interventions are tailored to individuals [3].

Despite its promise, the PM journey in Ontario encounters various hurdles, as highlighted by a recent study conducted by our team (Zavar, 2022) [2]. The healthcare system faces challenges due to inconsistent data governance across different health system levels and the complexity of federal and provincial acts such as PHIPA and FIPPA. These challenges are compounded by the lack of data-sharing agreements, which results in information blockages. Within organizations, intricate privacy rules

---

[1] Corresponding author: Abbas Zavar, abbas.zavar@utoronto.ca

further complicate data sharing and management. Furthermore, there are noticeable gaps in record linkage and data interoperability, alongside inconsistencies in data standards. The system also grapples with data capture, access, and overall quality deficiencies. These issues are magnified by challenges in managing big data and the inadequacy of the current IT infrastructure [2].

The obstacles faced extend beyond just data creation, dissemination, and preservation. They also delve into areas of policy formulation, innovation, and digital healthcare advancements. Such barriers underscore the prevalent issue of essential data being kept isolated and not being shared. Furthermore, there appears to be a lack of alignment in policy design, innovative efforts, and the progression of digital healthcare solutions—elements that are crucial for an effective PM strategy [2,4,5].

As one of Canada's most populous provinces, Ontario's healthcare infrastructure significantly influences the national landscape, and the potential of PM to redefine healthcare in this province is vast. Yet, to tap into this potential, a synchronized, comprehensive, and well-strategized approach is imperative.

2. Discussion

Designing a framework for PM necessitates a holistic approach that views PM as an intricate ecosystem. Just as every element within a natural ecosystem is interconnected and can positively or negatively influence one another, the PM domain functions similarly. Within the PM ecosystem, various elements - from healthcare professionals and policymakers to socioeconomic factors and technology providers - are all intertwined. Their individual actions and decisions reverberate throughout the system, having cascading effects on every other component. This interconnectedness underscores the importance of developing a comprehensive PM framework that does not just focus on the internal mechanics of healthcare but also factors in external influences.

A PM framework is a dynamic set of principles and strategies for the complex field of Precision Medicine. It is an adaptable guide that integrates scientific, technological, regulatory, and ethical considerations to enhance patient care and support the health community. Adopting this ecosystem viewpoint, the PM framework is crafted to be adaptive, resilient, and capable of aligning various elements to enhance patient care and benefit the health community at large [6,7].

The urgency for a PM framework arises from numerous challenges within the medical ecosystem. It highlights the critical need for cohesive leadership and harmonized policy-making. Here's a deep dive into the pivotal roles the framework seeks to serve:

- Guidance for System Leaders: PM is fast becoming the front-runner in healthcare advancement. For system leaders, it is essential to adapt to the financial aspects of implementing precision approaches, notably in areas like genomic sequencing and data analysis. They must focus on bridging the gap between conventional treatments and cutting-edge technologies to ensure equitable access to healthcare [8].
- Policy-making Tool: PM presents unique challenges that necessitate evidence-based policies. Implementing these policies should be backed by robust data and address current challenges, such as evidence gaps and an unprepared workforce, to ensure effective execution [9].

- A Beacon for Digital Health Developers: With the promise of enhanced outcomes, especially for chronic diseases, digital health solutions can be at the forefront of revolutionizing patient care. The key lies in these tools' rapid development and deployment, thus ensuring patients benefit from speed-to-market innovations [10].
- Resource for Researchers: PM is not just for a select few. There is a need to debunk misconceptions and understand that precision approaches have the potential to impact a broad patient demographic. Researchers can play a pivotal role by focusing on inclusive studies that cater to diverse patient populations [11].
- Framework for Pharmaceuticals: The path to harnessing the full potential of PM is laden with obstacles, from ethical dilemmas to data security. Pharmaceuticals must focus on agile governance and processes that adapt to these challenges while ensuring patient care remains at the center of their pursuits [12].
- Agile Governance in PM: Implementing an agile governance process that can improve government coordination, utilize public-private partnerships, and foster a nimble approach in the rapidly evolving PM field [12].

3.   Recommendations

- Develop a Comprehensive PM Framework: Emphasizing a holistic approach to PM, a strategic plan should encompass every element of the PM ecosystem. This includes elements both within and external to healthcare. Effective integration ensures that policies across various levels are harmonized, leadership strategies align coherently, innovations are coordinated, and standards for data, regulations, and other essential components are consistently met [13, 14]. Also, it is essential to have a well-defined and efficient strategy that captures the full scope of PM, integrating genetic, genomic, clinical, environmental, lifestyle and SDoH data [3].
- Invest in Data Infrastructure: To facilitate the progression of PM, embrace the potential of recent technological breakthroughs, such as artificial intelligence and blockchain technologies. These tools promise robust data collection, secure storage, and in-depth analysis capabilities [15,16].
- Digital Health Solution Innovation: A well-structured PM framework is a foundational guide for PM, stimulating innovation in digital health. It provides solution developers with a clear roadmap, emphasizing seamless integration and reducing redundancy, ensuring the inter-compatibility of digital health solutions. Furthermore, a cohesive framework promotes developers' adoption of uniform standards, leading to consistent user experiences across various platforms, whether for patients or healthcare professionals [17,18].
- Digital Health Policy Layer: The digital health policy layer is crucial for aligning the PM ecosystem with existing norms and regulations. A competent PM framework ensures regulatory compliance, prioritizes patient data privacy and security, and integrates advanced cybersecurity measures. It also addresses ethical concerns related to data usage and gains trust by emphasizing stakeholder engagement and promoting transparency in data

management practices. This comprehensive approach ensures widespread acceptance and confidence in digital health solutions [19-21].

- Data Governance and Advanced AI Implementation: A holistic PM approach demands the management and utilization of extensive data characterized by the various "Vs" of big data, including Volume, Velocity, Variety, Veracity, and Value. Effective handling of these datasets necessitates a rigorous data governance framework that guarantees data quality, security, and usability, as well as a detailed framework of data architecture covering all aspects, from data lakes to ETL processes [22].

Simultaneously, to tap into big data's potential, introducing advanced AI algorithms is pivotal. These AI solutions must be harmonized, integrated, and designed to work across platforms collaboratively. It's imperative for these AI algorithms to undergo rigorous training and validation processes to mitigate biases and errors. Ensuring an ethical deployment that refrains from inadvertent discrimination or decisions jeopardizing patient care is also fundamental for an inclusive PM strategy [17,20].

Incorporating these recommendations into the PM framework will not only facilitate the creation of a more holistic and patient-centric ecosystem but will also foster trust and collaboration among stakeholders in the digital health domain. By focusing strategically on big data management and the ethical and efficient implementation of AI solutions, the PM framework can ensure that healthcare solutions are both cutting-edge and trustable.

4. Conclusion

From Reactive to Proactive: In today's rapidly evolving medical landscape, a mere reactionary stance is no longer sufficient. A genuinely patient-centric system is not just about addressing immediate concerns or implementing short-lived interventions. It is about foreseeing future needs, understanding the broader context of healthcare, and crafting long-term strategies. The philosophy of Precision Medicine exemplifies this forward-thinking mindset. Instead of a narrow focus, PM demands a holistic perspective integrating genetic, environmental, lifestyle and SDoH factors to offer tailored healthcare solutions. To truly harness the potential of PM, we must proactively channel our resources, ensuring every tool, technology, and talent is oriented towards a unified vision. This involves creating a detailed and cohesive framework for the PM ecosystem, ensuring all components work harmoniously towards enhancing patient outcomes and advancing medical science.

References

[1] Ontario Health. OH Business Plan 2022-23 [Internet]. 2022 [cited 2023 Sep 23]. Available from: https://www.ontariohealth.ca/sites/ontariohealth/files/2022-05/OHBusinessPlan22_23.pdf

[2] Zavar A, Keshavjee K, Ling S, Brown E, Lalani M, Hussain A, et al. Preparing for Precision Medicine in Ontario: A Current State Assessment A report evaluating Ontario's current data sources and infrastructure to implement Precision Medicine initiatives [Internet]. Available from: https://www.canhealth.com/wp-content/uploads/2022/06/Precision-Medicine-Assessment-in-Ontario_May28.pdf

[3] Collins FS, Varmus H. A new initiative on precision medicine. N Engl J Med. 2015;372(9):793-5.

[4]   Government of Canada I. Unlocking the power of health data [Internet]. ised-isde.canada.ca. 2022. Available from: https://ised-isde.canada.ca/site/competition-bureau-canada/en/unlocking-power-health-data

[5]   RISING TO THE CHALLENGE FOR CANADA 2022-23 ANNUAL REPORT [Internet]. [cited 2023 Sep 23]. Available from: https://genomecanada.ca/wp-content/uploads/2023/07/GC-AnnualReport-2022-23_EN_web-2.pdf

[6]   Stenzinger A, Moltzen EK, Winkler E, Molnar-Gabor F, Malek N, Costescu A, et al. Implementation of precision medicine in healthcare-A European perspective. Journal of Internal Medicine [Internet]. 2023 Oct 1 [cited 2023 Sep 23];294(4):437–54. Available from: https://pubmed.ncbi.nlm.nih.gov/37455247/

[7]   Qoronfleh MW, Chouchane L, Mifsud B, Al Emadi M, Ismail S. THE FUTURE OF MEDICINE, healthcare innovation through precision medicine: policy case study of Qatar. Life Sciences, Society and Policy [Internet]. 2020 Nov 1;16. Available from: https://www.ncbi.nlm.nih.gov/pmc/articles/PMC7603723/

[8]   Precision Medicine: Challenges and Benefits [Internet]. Vicert. [cited 2023 Sep 23]. Available from: https://www.vicert.com/blog/precision-medicine

[9]   Naithani N, Atal AT, Tilak TVSVGK, Vasudevan B, Misra P, Sinha S. Precision medicine: Uses and challenges. Medical Journal Armed Forces India. 2021 Jul;77(3):258–65.

[10] Collaborations P, Europe, Focus G, America N. Precision Medicine: New Paradigms, Risks and Opportunities [Internet]. Knowledge@Wharton. Available from: https://knowledge.wharton.upenn.edu/article/precision-medicine-new-paradigms-risks-opportunities/

[11] Delivering large-scale patient impact through precision medicine [Internet]. STAT. [cited 2023 Sep 24]. Available from: https://www.statnews.com/sponsor/2023/06/14/delivering-large-scale-patient-impact-through-precision-medicine/

[12] Advancing precision medicine through agile governance [Internet]. Brookings. [cited 2023 Sep 24]. Available from: https://www.brookings.edu/articles/advancing-precision-medicine-through-agile-governance/

[13] Privy Council Office. Report to the Clerk of the Privy Council: A Data Strategy Roadmap for the Federal Public Service - Canada.ca [Internet]. Canada.ca. 2019. Available from: https://www.canada.ca/en/privy-council/corporate/clerk/publications/data-strategy.html

[14] 1.Secretariat TB of C. Digital Operations Strategic Plan: 2021–2024 [Internet]. www.canada.ca. 2021. Available from: https://www.canada.ca/en/government/system/digital-government/government-canada-digital-operations-strategic-plans/digital-operations-strategic-plan-2021-2024.html

[15] Seymour CW, Gomez H, Chang CCH, Clermont G, Kellum JA, Kennedy J, et al. Precision medicine for all? Challenges and opportunities for a precision medicine approach to critical illness. Critical Care. 2017 Oct 18;21(1).

[16] HealthITAnalytics. Top 3 Challenges of Integrating Precision Medicine with Routine Care [Internet]. HealthITAnalytics. 2020. Available from: https://healthitanalytics.com/news/top-3-challenges-of-integrating-precision-medicine-with-routine-care

[17] Abernethy A, Adams L, Barrett M, Bechtel C, Brennan P, Butte A, et al. The Promise of Digital Health: Then, Now, and the Future. NAM Perspectives. 2022 Jun 27;6(22).

[18] Poonsuph R. The Design Blueprint for a Large-Scale Telehealth Platform. Hu F, editor. International Journal of Telemedicine and Applications. 2022 Jan 5;2022:1–15.

[19] WHO. Draft global strategy on digital health 2020- 2025 GLOBAL STRATEGY ON DIGITAL HEALTH [Internet]. 2021. Available from: https://www.who.int/docs/default-source/documents/gs4dhdaa2a9f352b0445bafbc79ca799dce4d.pdf

[20] Digital Health Blueprint: Enabling Coordinated & Collaborative Health Care | Canada Health Infoway [Internet]. www.infoway-inforoute.ca. [cited 2023 Sep 24]. Available from: https://www.infoway-inforoute.ca/en/component/edocman/resources/technical-documents/architecture/2944-digital-health-blueprint-enabling-coordinated-collaborative-health-care?Itemid=103

[21] Precision Medicine Readiness Principles Resource Guide: Innovation Loop O C T O B E R 2 0 2 0 [Internet]. [cited 2023 Sep 24]. Available from: https://www3.weforum.org/docs/WEF_Resource_Guide_Innovation_Loop_2020.pdf

[22] Innovating Digital Health Solutions [Internet]. Ontario Centre of Innovation. [cited 2023 Sep 24]. Available from: https://www.oc-innovation.ca/programs/innovating-digital-health-solutions/

The Role of Digital Health Policy and Leadership
K. Keshavjee and A. Khatami (Eds.)
doi:10.3233/SHTI231307

From Blueprint to Best Practice: Gauging the Efficacy of Digital Health Solutions

Abbas ZAVAR [a1] and Razieh POORANDY [a]

[a] *Institute of Health Policy, Management and Evaluation, Dalla Lana School of Public Health, University of Toronto, Toronto, ON, Canada*
ORCiD ID: Abbas Zavar *https://orcid.org/0000-0003-0639-2765*

Abstract. The surge of AI-driven technologies in the digital health market demands a concurrent evolution in evaluation standards, a pace currently lagging behind innovation. This paper explores the pivotal inadequacies within existing evaluation models, highlighting the necessity for refined methodologies that align with the unique complexities of digital health. We critically examine the initiatives of key entities such as Health Canada, CADTH, and CNDHE, pinpointing the deficiencies in addressing the volatility and intricacies of AI applications. To bridge these gaps, we advocate for a nuanced evaluation paradigm, proposing the establishment of an oversight body, implementing detailed category-specific criteria, and a robust six-step evaluation framework tailored for AI health solutions. The paper culminates by underscoring the indispensable role of strategic leadership and agile policymaking in cultivating a resilient digital health environment that prioritizes patient care without compromising the ingenuity of technological advances.

Keywords. Digital health solutions, evaluation, AI-driven solutions, policymaking, standards

1. Introduction

The Digital Health sector has witnessed an exponential surge over the past two decades, introducing myriad innovations to the healthcare landscape. By 2030, projections forecast the global digital health market to reach an astounding $1.5 trillion [1]. Yet, a discernible contrast emerges as we move closer to this future. The rapid progression of these digital solutions, especially those powered by artificial intelligence, significantly outpaces the development of a standardized evaluation framework.

Historically, medical interventions have undergone rigorous evaluations, ensuring they meet stringent standards before introduction to the marketplace. However, with their unique attributes, digital health solutions present an entirely different set of challenges than their traditional counterparts. Recognizing these disparities, international regulatory bodies have made attempts to categorize these digital innovations, coining terms such as "Software as a Medical Device" (SaMD) in the US and "Medical Device Software" (MDSW) in the EU. Despite these categorizations, a substantial portion of these tools remains unsupported by tangible evidence confirming their clinical claims [2,3].

As the number of applications continues to rise, the methodologies for their timely, cost-effective, and robust evaluations lag behind. Current frameworks have failed to adapt to the diverse nature of these solutions, with each category requiring distinct

---

[1] Corresponding author: Abbas Zavar, abbas.zavar@utoronto.ca

evaluation criteria [2]. This has given rise to a conspicuous gap where developers are left without standardized creation guidelines, end-users, including physicians, are devoid of comparative standards, and researchers grapple with the absence of unified efficacy evaluation criteria for these digital health tools. The resulting scenario paints a worrisome picture; an overflow of digital health solutions, with a glaring disconnect between their sheer quantity and proven quality.

Artificial Intelligence (AI) rapidly transforms the healthcare industry by offering innovative solutions to complex problems. AI solutions in healthcare are increasingly vital for their capacity to address current challenges and their role in shaping the future of medicine and public health. The intersection of AI with healthcare promises revolutionary breakthroughs, but the absence of a coherent evaluation system threatens this potential. Without clear, universally accepted standards, there lies an inherent risk of compromising the efficacy of these Digital Health Solutions (DHS). Stakeholders, whether patients, healthcare providers, or developers, require transparent and standardized evaluation mechanisms to navigate this burgeoning digital landscape. Without these mechanisms, they remain at risk of sifting through myriad solutions, many of which might be unverified or ineffective, making the pressing need for a comprehensive evaluation system for digital health, particularly AI-enabled solutions, undeniable.

The following sections of this paper will delve into the current state of evaluation mechanisms, identifying their limitations and proposing a focused framework specifically tailored to address the complexities inherent in AI-driven digital health solutions.

2.   Discussion

2.1 Health Canada

A leading health institution in the nation launched its "Guidance Document: Software as a Medical Device (SaMD): Definition and Classification" in 2019, focusing on the intricate digital health realm. This guidance delivers a clear categorization system based on SaMD's purpose and employs a risk-based approach, effectively evaluating higher-risk software and including AI-integrated SaMDs [4].

The guidance may seem limited in scope, overlooking emerging digital health tech. It might be perceived as leaning heavily towards established medical models, possibly neglecting patient-centric innovations and data management advancements. The lack of emphasis on data privacy, system interoperability, and user interface is also concerning. Issues arise in the AI context. The dynamic behaviour of AI is not addressed, nor are transparency concerns, data bias, or continuous AI validation. Furthermore, the guidance does not cater to AI's vulnerability to adversarial attacks, interactions with other AI systems, or the challenge of generalizing AI models across varied datasets or populations. Thus, while valuable, the guidance requires a more in-depth perspective on AI's challenges in healthcare [4].

2.2. Canadian Agency for Drugs and Technologies in Health (CADTH)

CADTH is an esteemed organization in Canada focusing on evaluating health technologies. One of its core sectors entails appraising digital health solutions (DHS).

Emphasizing this mission, CADTH pioneered the establishment of Canada's First Digital Health Evaluation Network, aiming to thoroughly examine digital health interventions' safety, efficacy, and value. By offering evidence-based insights into digital health, CADTH ensures that stakeholders and policymakers are updated with the latest digital health advancements and methodologies [5].

Critically, while CADTH recognizes the importance of DHS, it lacks specificity regarding its approaches or guidelines, especially concerning AI-enabled solutions. This paucity of detailed information makes it difficult to thoroughly critique their role in the digital health domain. Although CADTH has shown signs of acknowledging the rapidly progressing field of AI in clinical applications, the exact ways in which they assess or endorse AI-powered solutions remain somewhat veiled. Additionally, their "Rapid Response Service" suggests a possible avenue for addressing pressing health technology inquiries, but its application to DHS or AI-specific concerns seems uncertain. In light of policy perspectives on health technologies becoming obsolete, CADTH does seem to indirectly grasp the need for perpetually refreshed evaluation standards in healthcare, yet concrete plans for DHS are still wanting.

2.3. Canadian Network for Digital Health Evaluation (CNDHE) and Centre for Digital Health Evaluation (CDHE)

CNDHE and CDHE are organizations driving the evaluation of digital health interventions across Canada. Positioned under Health Canada's jurisdiction, they aim to form a comprehensive strategy for digital health evaluation. This effort's main objective is the creation of the Pan-Canadian Digital Health Evaluation Framework. This framework aims to give researchers a unified blueprint for evaluations, grounded in significant research and collaboration, and is captured in a Conceptual Model with stages of Planning, Implementing, and Impact, aiming to foster a Learning Health System [6].

However, the model's broader scope may be its downfall. It lacks detailed instructions for varied digital health solutions, making practical application challenging. Concerns arise around its flexibility to accommodate emergent themes and clarity about stakeholder involvement. For AI solutions, the model must emphasize Explainable AI (XAI) for transparency, integrate ethical guidelines considering fairness, biases, and privacy, and consider interaction dynamics between humans and AI. It should also consider the continuous learning nature of AI, the importance of diverse training datasets, and the educational impact on health professionals [6].

3. Recommendations

To navigate the complex interplay between standardization and innovation in AI-enabled digital health solutions, our recommendations advocate for a balanced, multi-faceted approach to evaluation. Recognizing the necessity for rigorous standards while also allowing for the dynamic nature of technological advancement, the following structured yet adaptable recommendations are proposed.

3.1. Establishment of a Dedicated Oversight Body

It is imperative to institute an independent oversight body to unify the evaluation standards. This entity will be responsible for establishing and updating uniform criteria tailored to the distinct categories of Digital Health Solutions (DHS), with special attention to the unique characteristics of AI-driven technologies. This approach ensures that each category is evaluated against relevant and stringent standards, thereby balancing rigorous evaluation and encouraging innovative development practices.

3.2. Adoption of Detailed and Category-Specific Standards

Categorical specificity ensures uniformity in development, leading to easier comparison and evaluation of products. Encourage developers and providers to adapt their production strategies according to meticulous criteria specific to each category. This not only standardizes the development process but also assists end-users in comparing and evaluating similar products within the same category.

3.3. Introduction of Burnout Evaluation

Considering the critical issue of physician burnout, we recommend the inclusion of evaluation criteria that specifically address the impact of DHS on healthcare providers. By assessing whether a tool alleviates or exacerbates burnout, we can better gauge its overall benefit to the healthcare system and its providers, thereby ensuring that the well-being of clinicians is a factor in the utility assessment of digital health innovations [7].

3.4. Implementation of a Comprehensive Six-Step Evaluation for AI Solutions

To assess AI solutions comprehensively, we endorse a structured six-step evaluation process that considers the following dimensions: (1) Initial alignment with healthcare needs, (2) Technical robustness, (3) Clinical outcome relevance, (4) User experience efficiency, (5) System integration capability, and (6) Ethical and privacy safeguards. This framework guarantees comprehensive assessments, covering practicality, clinical efficacy, and alignment with recognized benchmarks. [8] This methodology does not intend to create redundancies with Health Technology Assessment (HTA) but rather to serve as a specific, actionable framework within the broader HTA context, addressing the unique demands of AI in healthcare.

3.5. Development of an Adaptive Evaluation Ecosystem

Acknowledging the fast-paced evolution of digital health, it is crucial to establish systematic and capable evaluation mechanisms to adjust to new developments. By implementing structures that are designed to be organized yet flexible, the evaluation process can remain up-to-date with the latest advancements, ensuring both the reliability and relevance of evaluations [9].

3.6 Integration of Health Technology Assessment (HTA) in Evaluation

HTA's well-established, comprehensive methodology for assessing the various impacts of health technologies is invaluable. By incorporating HTA into the broader evaluation framework, we ensure a thorough understanding of a technology's potential impacts. This integration allows for informed policy and decision-making that fully accounts for health technology's medical, social, economic, and ethical dimensions [10].

4. Conclusion

Fueled by the digital revolution, the evolution toward a proactive healthcare framework marks a critical juncture in health service delivery. It brings to the fore the essential requirement for robust evaluation methods that are specifically designed for AI-driven digital health solutions. While there are concerted efforts to devise comprehensive evaluation systems, the heterogeneity of digital health solutions demands nuanced, category-specific assessment tools.

Evaluation now transcends clinical efficacy, including user engagement, ethical data management, and technological congruence within healthcare systems. Therefore, an effective evaluation framework must marry traditional healthcare assessment with the novel complexities introduced by AI technologies.

As we transition to a proactive healthcare model, our evaluative practices must also evolve, incorporating both established and emerging research methods that reflect the agility of digital health advancements. This integrated approach ensures relevance and drives innovation within the sector.

Leadership and policymaking play pivotal roles in this shift. Visionaries championing adaptive evaluation models and policymakers supporting their widespread implementation are indispensable for establishing a robust digital health ecosystem.

Provided recommendations advocate for an evaluation environment that judiciously combines rigor and flexibility. This approach seeks to uphold the integrity and utility of digital health innovations, paving the way for a healthcare landscape where safety, efficacy, and innovation are harmoniously balanced for the betterment of patient care.

References

[1]   Research and Markets. Digital Health Market Size, Share & Trends Analysis Report. [Internet]. [Date unknown] [cited 2023 Sep 17]. Available from: https://www.researchandmarkets.com/reports/5265093/digital-health-market-size-share-and-trends

[2]   Guo C, Ashrafian H, Ghafur S, Fontana G, Gardner C, Prime M. Challenges for the evaluation of digital health solutions—A call for innovative evidence generation approaches. NPJ Digital Medicine. 2020;3(1):1-14. Available from: https://doi.org/10.1038/s41746-020-00314-2

[3]   The SAMD Regulatory Landscape in the US and EU. Regulatory Affairs Professionals Society. Published August 23, 2021. Accessed September 17, 2023. Available from: https://www.raps.org/news-and-articles/news-articles/2021/8/the-samd-regulatory-landscape-in-the-us-and-eu-1

[4]   Health Canada. Software as a Medical Device (SAMD) Guidance Document. Accessed September 17, 2023. Available from: https://www.canada.ca/en/health-canada/services/drugs-health-products/medical-devices/application-information/guidance-documents/software-medical-device-guidance-document.html

[5]   CADTH. Collaboration in Health Technology Assessment in Canada. https://www.cadth.ca/collaboration-health-technology-assessment-canada [Accessed September 17, 2023].

[6]   Women's College Hospital. Conceptual Model. https://cndhe.womenscollegehospital.ca/network/conceptual-model/ [Accessed September 17, 2023].

[7]   Zavar A, Ling S, Chandrasena C, Han J, Fahey-Walsh J. Physician Burnout: Potential Causes & Solutions. Available from: https://www.ontariomd.ca/documents/resource%20library/ontariomd-physician-burnout-brochure-aug-2%20final.pdf [Accessed September 17, 2023].

[8]   Mathews S, Prime MS. Evaluating digital health solutions: How to know which solutions will bring value to your organization? [Internet]. Available from: https://healthcaretransformers.com/digital-health/current-trends/evaluating-digital-health-solutions-event/ [Accessed 17 September 2023].

[9]   Ghafur S, Prime MS. New approaches to evaluate digital solutions with clinical value. [Internet]. Available from: https://healthcaretransformers.com/digital-health/current-trends/evaluating-digital-health-solutions-clinical-value/ [Accessed 17 September 2023].

[10] World Health Organization. Health Technology Assessment and Health Benefit Package Survey 2020/2021. https://www.who.int/teams/health-systems-governance-and-financing/economic-analysis/health-technology-assessment-and-benefit-package-design/survey-homepage [Accessed 17 September 2023].

The Role of Digital Health Policy and Leadership
K. Keshavjee and A. Khatami (Eds.)
© 2024 The Authors.
This article is published online with Open Access by IOS Press and distributed under the terms
of the Creative Commons Attribution Non-Commercial License 4.0 (CC BY-NC 4.0).
doi:10.3233/SHTI231308

Implementation of a Clinical, Patient-Level Dashboard at a Mental Health Hospital: Lessons Learned from Two Pilot Clinics

Masooma HASSAN[a,c1], Jose Arturo SANTISTEBAN[a,b] and Nelson SHEN[b,c]

aCentre for Addiction and Mental Health, Toronto, ON, Canada, Institute of Health Policy, Management and Evaluation, University of Toronto, Toronto, ON, Canada
bKrembil Centre for Neuroinformatics, Centre for Addiction and Mental Health, Toronto, ON, Canada
cInstitute of Health Policy, Management and Evaluation, University of Toronto, Dalla Lana School of Public Health, Toronto, ON, Canada

ORCID: Masooma Hassan https://orcid.org/0000-0001-6185-5051, Jose Arturo Santisteban https://orcid.org/0000-0002-4109-984X, Nelson Shen https://orcid.org/0000-0003-1788-8176

Abstract. The Centre for Addiction and Mental Health has implemented mechanisms to standardize routine data collection with the vision of a Learning Health System. To improve clinical decision-making and patient outcomes, a clinical dashboard was implemented to provide a real-time visualization of data from patient self-assessments and other physical and mental health indicators. This case report shares early findings of dashboard implementation to understand user uptake and improve fidelity of the technology and processes that need to support adoption. Moreover, these findings will inform the strategy and development of a hospital-wide scalable dashboard that will span across clinical areas and leverage artificial intelligence to continuously improve patient outcomes and equitable care delivery.

Keywords. Clinical dashboard, learning health system, implementation, mental health, digital

1. Introduction

A Learning Health System (LHS) is a data-driven approach in which research, data, and experiences are continuously collected to iteratively and recursively innovate and improve healthcare practices, processes, and policies—all with the objective of improving patient outcomes and equitable healthcare delivery. The backbone of the LHS is a strong health data infrastructure which leverages information technology to systematically capture and analyze data and care experiences and apply this evidence in real-time to guide care. At the clinic-level, this real-time data can be accessed by clinicians and patients through clinical dashboards to support timely, informed, and evidence-based decisions about treatments; moreover, the integration of data science and genomics will enable personalized and precision medicine, thereby enabling tailored treatments based on predictive modelling and risk stratification. The LHS and

---

[1][1] Corresponding Author: Masooma Hassan, masooma.hassan@camh.ca

precision medicine are quickly becoming a reality with the ongoing digital transformation of healthcare and the rapid advancements in digital technology and data analytics [1].

In 2018, the Centre for Addiction and Mental Health (CAMH) started to lay the foundation for a LHS by providing a framework for continuous data collection and for measuring the impact of changes. As the largest academic mental health hospital in Canada, CAMH has developed and implemented 24 integrated care pathways (ICPs). ICPs enable the use of structured evidence-based care plans to provide standardized and improved patient care for the 34,000 patients they support annually. Through the ICPs, CAMH implemented Measurement-Based Care (MBC), a process in which patients complete self-assessments at regular intervals. The routine collection of data allows for the tracking of a patient's progress and response to treatment over time. At CAMH, the data is collected digitally through a clinical instance of REDCap—a free secure web-application for building and managing electronic surveys and assessments. The REDCap data is then automatically transferred to the CAMH-branded Cerner Millennium Electronic Health Record, I-CARE. Together, these mechanisms allow CAMH to collect, streamline and leverage patient information to enhance clinical decision-making and give patients agency in their recovery process [2]. Clinical dashboards were implemented to provide clinicians' access to this rich dataset.

Clinical dashboards provide clinicians with timely access to multiple sources of routinely collected data in a visual, concise, and user-friendly format. Clinical dashboards have been found to facilitate effective access of information, improve communications and information sharing, and support clinical decision-making [3]. To enable this, I-CARE was integrated with Tableau data visualization software to provide a personalized holistic data visualization of a patient's care journey directly within the patient's chart. This novel approach allows clinicians to customize and review patient trajectory information such as assessment scores, medication trajectory, appointment indicators, and other types of indicators and information. Clinicians were engaged throughout the development process interface design, data validation, and dashboard testing to ensure the dashboard met their needs. The "Tool+Team+Routine" heuristic [4] was used as a way to understand the dashboard (Tool), clinical perspectives on value (Team), and integration into workflows (Routine). This service design strategy is intended to optimize the value of the dashboard to its users. To this end, a clinical champion model was also implemented to sustain clinical engagement, support the implementation, and enable clinician-driven evolution of the dashboard. Clinical champions were identified and took the role of a 'super user', tailoring and facilitating the training and onboarding their clinics. Routine touchpoints with the clinical champions allowed the project team to monitor and optimize the dashboard based on feedback from their clinics; however, open communications channels enabled feedback and report backs between touchpoints.

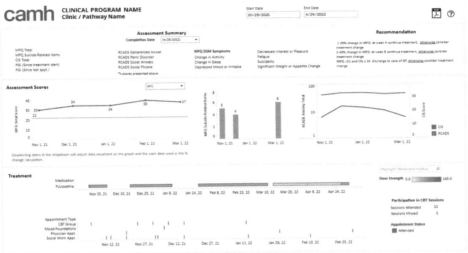

Figure 1. Clinical Dashboard User Interface.

This case report provides the lessons learned from the pilot implementation of clinical dashboards in two clinics that were implemented in the first quarter of 2022 / 2023. These clinics use an MBC approach with patients. The dashboard users consist of physicians, nurses, and allied health professionals in the Ontario Structured Psychotherapy program (OSP) and CARIBOU-ICP. The OSP provides cognitive-behavioral therapy (CBT) and/or a related approach to treating patients with depression, anxiety, and anxiety-related conditions. The CARIBOU-ICP is a structured, multi-disciplinary, and collaborative approach in assessing and monitoring their progress in youth with depression.

2. Methods

Given the early stage maturity of the CAMH clinical dashboards, a process monitoring approach was undertaken to continuously understand how the intervention is being implemented (i.e., fidelity). This process was supported by monitoring back-end analytics and routine engagement via the Clinical Champions Model. Back-end analytics were used to identify use patterns across the two clinics. Based on Proctors' Implementation Outcomes [5], the metrics reported here include adoption (i.e., # users, #views), penetrance (# users/total clinicians), and feasibility (average # views/user). The back-end analytics served as a foundation for engaging the clinical champions, where their feedback provided context to the identified trends.

Starting at two months post-implementation, the project team met with the clinical champion from each clinic separately at approximately 3-month intervals. The objective of the meetings was to understand the clinical experiences with the dashboard, provide dashboard updates, and discuss feedback gathered by the clinical champions. The purpose of the meetings were to identify ways to improve fidelity of the clinic implementation. This paper reports on the key findings from these discussions.

3. Results

3.1. Back-end Analytics

Between May 2022 to September 2023, the dashboard was viewed 270 times in the OSP Clinic and had a penetrance of 50.0% (16/32 clinicians). In terms of feasibility, the dashboard was viewed 16.8 times/user; (range 1-67). The dashboard was viewed 80 times by the CARIBOU clinic and had a penetrance of 83.3% (5/6 clinicians). In terms of feasibility, the dashboard was viewed 16.0 times/user (range 1-55).

3.2. Feedback from clinical champion engagement

Eleven meetings were held with the clinical champions over 17 months. While most of the meeting focused on understanding the usefulness of the dashboard, the following are overarching feedback related to the clinical dashboard use.

Perceived usefulness: When discussing how the dashboard was useful, there was positive feedback mostly around the ability to have visualized data, in that it was a quick way to visually assess patients' symptoms over time. Clinicians found it helpful to have the dashboard available to view treatment progress over time or during the time of discharge to complete discharge summaries. The pilot sites demanded the need for more patient-level clinical dashboards across each outpatient area.

Adaptation to workflow: CARIBOU clinic mentioned that they use the dashboard in team meetings, in a group setting to inform clinical care. The team used the dashboard to view patient trajectory and discuss aspects of clinical care together. Some clinicians also shared it with the patient to discuss treatment trajectory together. In OSP, clinicians use the dashboard right before their appointment with the client, or during the appointment.

Training and Awareness: There was a need to improve digital literacy for using the dashboard as many clinicians expressed the need for more training as some forgot how to access or use it. Other clinicians did not understand the purpose of the dashboard or forgot it existed.

Technology limitations: Lack of real-time data availability on the dashboard inhibited the clinicians from using the dashboard. Especially in the case where the dashboard was viewed soon after the patient completed assessments (in some cases, five minutes after). Variations in processes across the organization affected the quality of data on the dashboard - if the data was not entered on time or if there was variation in data entry workflow across an area, this impacted the availability of the data on the dashboard thereby not providing a complete picture to the clinicians.

4. Discussion and Conclusion

Based on the metrics presented here, the clinical dashboards were implemented with slow success. The barriers to adoption could be attributed to the technological challenges of using the dashboard and the lag in the real-time data, both limiting its value to its users. Moreover, the dashboard did not make a strong impression as many clinicians did not remember it and did not know why they should be using it. With the limited capacity of the workforce and the competing priorities, this finding suggests that continuing efforts should be made to engage clinicians to understand how we can increase the dashboards' relevance and bring value to their practice and patient outcomes [6].

Despite the low adoption, there were some lessons learned that can be used to support clinical adoption of these tools. Some clinicians in both the OSP and CARIBOU clinic perceived the usefulness or value of having the dashboard to inform clinical decision-making. The CARIBOU clinic found value in a workflow that was not as originally anticipated: the dashboard was used individually by the clinicians during the time of the appointment with the patient. The CARIBOU clinic adapted the dashboard workflow by using it in team meetings to discuss patient progress and to co-develop a treatment plan. These adaptations drove adoption and usage, echoing the "Tool+Team+Routine" heuristic, where its alignment between these three factors created a strong value proposition for the clinics [4]. While this case report contributes to the growing literature on dashboard implementation, these reflections are intended to share some lessons learned from the clinical champions and the implementation experience. These interim insights will need to be validated through an evaluation. A formative mixed-method evaluation will be conducted to improve the dashboard experience at the pilot clinics and guide implementation in other clinics. The evaluation will take a developmental and participatory approach, where clinicians will be iteratively engaged to optimize the dashboard value and define success, especially given the different workflows for the two sites.

This experience highlighted the importance of continued engagement with the clinical champions. This process is essential in ensuring that mechanisms are in place for quickly fixing dashboard features to support utility and adoption. More importantly, this keeps clinicians continuously engaged in the monitoring process. Low engagement from clinical users resulted in more difficulty in gathering insights on adoption barriers and supporting the clinical teams in addressing barriers. Sustained engagement will be vital to the development and implementation of a scalable dashboard across all clinical areas at CAMH—a project driven by clinician feedback. This work stream includes the integration of complex, interacting factors in the ICP data with machine learning to generate meaningful predictive insights, such as which patients are likely to improve on certain treatments or which patients may be at risk for suicide. While CAMH policies and procedures for data collection through the MBC and ICPs create the foundational infrastructure, other organizational policies and processes will be required to support this end. As presented in the feedback, data availability, data entry, and data quality are factors that would impact the value of the dashboard. The lack of quality data would further impact the ability to develop unbiased and accurate machine learning outputs [7]. Furthermore, system-level policies will be required to close the loop by feeding back the results of analyses of the data collected to the clinic that collected the original data, thereby enabling the continuous improvement approach of a LHS. These policies and procedures will need to be part of any machine learning or AI models that need continuous refinement and improvement to prevent drift (i.e., reduction in accuracy over time). The vision is for the generated knowledge or models created by the LHS to be communicated or applied through clinical-decision support dashboards.

References

[1] Lim HC, Austin JA, van der Vegt AH, Rahimi AK, Canfell OJ, Mifsud J, et al. Toward a Learning Health Care System: A Systematic Review and Evidence-Based Conceptual Framework for Implementation of Clinical Analytics in a Digital Hospital. Appl Clin Inform. 2022 Mar;13(2):339-354. doi: 10.1055/s-0042-1743243.

[2] Hawley S, Yu J, Bogetic N, Potapova N, Wakefield C, Thompson M, et al. Digitization of Measurement-Based Care Pathways in Mental Health Through REDCap and Electronic Health Record Integration: Development and Usability Study. J Med Internet Res. 2021 May 20;23(5):e25656. doi: 10.2196/25656.

[3] Dowding D, Randell R, Gardner P, Fitzpatrick G, Dykes P, Favela J, et al. Dashboards for improving patient care: review of the literature. Int J Med Inform. 2015 Feb;84(2):87-100. doi: 10.1016/j.ijmedinf.2014.10.001.

[4] Shaw J, Agarwal P, Desveaux L, Palma DC, Stamenova V, Jamieson T, Yang R, Bhatia RS, Bhattacharyya O. Beyond "implementation": digital health innovation and service design. NPJ Digit Med. 2018 Sep 20;1:48. doi: 10.1038/s41746-018-0059-8.

[5] Proctor E, Silmere H, Raghavan R, Hovmand P, Aarons G, Bunger A, Griffey R, Hensley M. Outcomes for implementation research: conceptual distinctions, measurement challenges, and research agenda. Adm Policy Ment Health. 2011 Mar;38(2):65-76. doi: 10.1007/s10488-010-0319-7.

[6] Jankovic I, Chen JH. Clinical Decision Support and Implications for the Clinician Burnout Crisis. Yearb Med Inform. 2020 Aug;29(1):145-154. doi: 10.1055/s-0040-1701986.

[7] Secinaro S, Calandra D, Secinaro A, Muthurangu V, Biancone P. The role of artificial intelligence in healthcare: a structured literature review. BMC Med Inform Decis Mak. 2021 Apr 10;21(1):125. doi: 10.1186/s12911-021-01488-9.

Regulation, Governance and Interoperability

The Role of Digital Health Policy and Leadership
K. Keshavjee and A. Khatami (Eds.)
doi:10.3233/SHTI231310

Towards a Unified Framework for Information and Interoperability Governance

Anna TUMULAK[a], Jennifer TIN[a] and Karim KESHAVJEE[a,1]
[a] *Institute of Health Policy, Management and Evaluation, Dalla Lana School of Public Health, University of Toronto, Toronto, ON, Canada*
ORCiD ID: Karim Keshavjee https://orcid.org/0000-0003-1317-7035

Abstract. Challenges in health data interoperability have highlighted overall health care system inefficiencies. Many organizations struggle to establish a robust data governance infrastructure to meet the increasing demands of advanced data uses, let alone sharing it with a large number of other organizations. There is a need for health care organizations to adopt information governance frameworks that encapsulates interoperability as a core attribute as this can improve data processing, knowledge translation and participation in the larger health data ecosystem. To establish interoperability between healthcare organizations, standards must exist in relation to how information is governed and circulates in the healthcare system, not just on how it is structured, stored and used within an organization. In this paper we demonstrate that interoperability between organizations cannot coherently exist without consideration of information governance within organizations. Lack of coherence can lead to lack of data accessibility, decreased organizational efficiencies, and poor data quality. With this in mind, we propose a unified framework that integrates the principles of both information and interoperability governance to increase the adaptability, flexibility, and efficiency of health information usage across the entire healthcare system.

Keywords. Information governance, data governance, interoperability governance

1. Introduction

Health data interoperability is becoming an increasingly urgent challenge in Canada's healthcare system, as many parts of the healthcare system have been computerized for over a decade [1]. However, many organizations struggle to establish a robust data governance infrastructure to meet the increasing demand of advanced data uses, let alone sharing it with large numbers of other organizations. As more than 80% of health care data are digitalized [1], there is a need for health care organizations to adopt data governance frameworks that incorporate interoperability as an important element that enhances the processing and translation of data for health system transformation. A robust data governance framework could lead to improved clinical decision making and reduced operational costs. However, challenges persist as data governance and interoperability are often considered to be separate entities. The most significant barrier

---

[1] Corresponding Author: Karim Keshavjee karim.keshavjee@utoronto.ca

to enhancing interoperability in health care systems is related to how data is governed and managed within organizations [2].

In today's rapidly evolving digital healthcare landscape, the application of artificial intelligence (AI) and machine learning (ML) to health care processes places even greater emphasis on the importance of how these technologies can produce insights and analytics more consistently [3]. To increase trust and value in these technologies, data governance and interoperability governance principles need to be integrated and aligned to meet business and operational goals. Through the process of developing the unified framework, we identified a key difference between data and information; information has meaning while data needs more context to have meaning. We therefore changed our focus from data governance to information governance to ensure that only meaningful information is shared between healthcare providers. With this in mind, we propose a framework that will integrate the principles of both information and interoperability governance to increase the adaptability, flexibility, and efficiency of health care and aid in health system transformation [2].

2.   Methods

We developed a set of requirements for information governance and interoperability based on the challenges faced by and the data needs of key stakeholders in the healthcare system, including patients, providers, payors, policymakers, researchers, data managers and administrators. These requirements drove the development of our framework. We reviewed a variety of existing data governance frameworks to identify components that could satisfy the requirements [4-6].

The unified framework was developed through an iterative process of selecting components that addressed the requirements and developing new requirements based on components found in the various frameworks that were relevant in the healthcare system. We iteratively revised the framework until no new requirements or components were identified. Based on extensive literature search in Google Scholar and PubMed, to our knowledge, this is the first study to focus on a unified information and interoperability governance (UIIG) framework.

3.   Challenges with Unified Information and Interoperability Governance

Some of the common challenges in information governance include access management, fragmented and siloed data, lack of resources, lack of training, and lack of professional accountability. All these challenges lead to poor clinical decision-making, decreased stakeholder efficiency, and an unsustainable digital health care landscape. To uphold the value of data assets, organizations need to carefully consider their approach to IIG.

As each health care organization uses varying health information systems, there is a need to recognize the importance of health information exchange, usability, and translation of clinical data. To establish interoperability between health systems, standards must exist in relation to how information is governed and cycles in health care organizations. Therefore, interoperability cannot exist without the consideration of information governance as it can lead to the lack of data accessibility, decreased organizational efficiencies, and poor data quality [7].

4. Requirements for a Unified IIG Framework

Table 1 lists the requirements identified by our team. Many of these requirements are discussed in a variety of digital discourses but are rarely listed in one place.

Table 1. List of stakeholder requirements.

Stakeholder	Requirements
All stakeholders	Collect once, use many; easily transformable for a variety of uses; easily accessible by authorized individuals; easily visualized; easy to act upon; high quality data
Patient	Improved safety; minimal loss of privacy; access to own data.
Policy-maker	Compliant with legislation; integrates with multiple EMRs; compatible with international standards.
Funder	Cost-effective; value for money.
Healthcare Provider	Not burdensome for entry or retrieval; access to knowledge bases; tools for risk profiling; compatible with multiple data entry forms; ability to share clinical data across institutions;
Administrator	Risk profiling; collect process data; value for money.
Researcher	Quick access to data; easily link to additional datasets (exposures, deprivation index, etc.); captures data from a variety of systems; ability to conduct controlled experiments.
Data manager	Tools for cleansing; statistical modeling and visualization.

5. Proposed Unified IIG Framework

The resulting combined information and interoperability governance framework is shown in Figure 1.

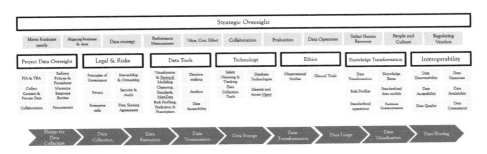

Figure 1. Proposed unified information and interoperability governance framework.

Strategic oversight is essential in the implementation of an effective unified information governance and interoperability framework across the health care system. This allows for organizations to align and secure data assets, conduct reviews, and monitor organizational goals, mission, and vision consistently and systematically. There are 11 elements identified within the strategic oversight layer of this framework. These include the following key drivers in achieving optimal strategic oversight: 1) Meet Business Needs, 2) Aligning Business & Data, 3) Sets Data Strategy, 4) Performance Measurement, 5) Optimize Value, Cost, Effort, 6) Collaboration, 7)

Evaluation, 8) Data Openness and FAIR compliance, 9) Skilled Human Resources, 10) People and Culture, 11) Regulating Vendors.

There are seven key components along with their associated operational requirements to establish a robust IIG program within any organization. The following is a brief description for each framework component:

- Project Data Oversight is foundational to the management of data collected, transmitted, stored, and used in projects within the organization and defines what processes, tools, and principles are required to achieve oversight.
- Legal and Risks should be considered as data is viewed as an asset and having value. It is also highly regulated in the healthcare sector.
- Data Tools needed for visualization and statistical modelling. Ensures value of data for all stakeholders is achieved. Can also be shared across the system.
- Technology for automating risk management wherever possible.
- Ethics assessment is necessary throughout each phase of the data pipeline to ensure organizations continually assess data practices and policies with a focus on how this impacts data owners and society. Ethics is required for research studies and to ensure AI used by the organization is unbiased.
- Knowledge transformation. Data should be easily transformable and produce meaningful and useful clinical, administrative, research, policy and resource allocation insights across all institutions.
- Interoperability. Information should be easily shared, utilized, and translated across systems. Focus should be on utility of information, not data transfer.

Below the framework key components and requirements is the data lifecycle layer. The data lifecycle identifies all the stages of the data lifecycle, which need to be governed, including the stage when the data collection and use is being contemplated and designed.

6.   Policy Options

Our healthcare system has three options with regards to information governance and interoperability governance. The first option is to continue to keep the two separate. This has the benefit of not having to invest in additional stakeholder engagement, redesign of governance frameworks and training for a new governance framework. The cons are that the current approach does not work and has not worked for many years, leading to fragmented data, poor performance and inability to share information effectively for patient care and provider effectiveness. Lack of unified governance will make it difficult to take advantage of new technologies like artificial intelligence and generative AI.

The second option is to create a shared health information governance framework [8] that creates a multi-stakeholder governance structure for overseeing the management of all data in the healthcare system. The benefits of this approach are appealing in a democratic setting where everyone contributes to identifying shared goals, identifying risks and then working together to oversee the tracking of information across the system. The key issues with this framework are that it is very difficult to operationalize and puts too much emphasis on the stakeholders and very little on the day-to-day operational aspects of IIG.

The third and recommended option is the Unified Information and Interoperability Governance (UIIG) framework whose benefits are that it codifies best practices, enables rapid updates across the system because everyone is on the same page and enables sharing of tools and methods across similar types of organizations. The issues with this framework are the high initial investment requirements in converting from current approaches to the new approach.

7. Benefits of a Unified IIG Framework

Adoption of a UIIG framework will enable organizations to promote operational efficiency and more readily comply with regulatory requirements. A unified framework will speed up training, onboarding and decision-making. It will also enable consistency, improve data quality, and improve decision-making within and across organizations. Additionally, it will set clear and standardized guidelines across the country which will increase efficiency in system-wide and organizational oversight as data is managed, governed, and exchanged according to similar guiding principles and concepts.

A unified framework will promote trust, security, and alignment of organizational goals. It will also enable sharing of best practices and tools that could speed up the adoption of the UIIG framework and lower the costs of interoperability.

8. Conclusion and Recommendations

For our healthcare system to become more proactive, actionable information needs to be available at key pivot points in a patient's health trajectory. Opportunities for proactive care, once lost, are lost forever and the patient is destined for heavy health system use. Our proposed UIIG framework could potentially enable safer and more efficient sharing of information across the healthcare system 1) without overwhelming patients with too many access points (or none at all), 2) without overwhelming healthcare providers with data that has more noise than signal, 3) making it easier to train and on-board employees and providers and 4) making it easier to share tools and best practices across the healthcare system. We highly recommend governments and key stakeholders consider adoption of the Unified Information and Interoperability Governance framework.

References

[1] Dong L, Keshavjee K. Why is information governance important for electronic healthcare systems? A Canadian experience. Journal of Advances in Humanities and Social Sciences. 2016 Oct;2(5):250-60.

[2] González L. Data Interoperability Guide. UN Statistics Wiki. 2018 Oct. Available at https://unstats.un.org/wiki/x/eoMnAg. Accessed Sept 11, 2023.

[3] Canadian Institute for Health Information. CIHI's Health Data and Information Governance and Capability Framework. Ottawa, ON: CIHI; 2020.

[4] Panian Z. Some practical experiences in data governance. World Academy of Science, Engineering and Technology. 2010 Oct;62(1):939-46.

[5] The Data Governance Institute. The DGI Data Governance Framework; 2023 [cited 2023 Sept 11]. Available from: https://datagovernance.com/the-dgi-data-governance-framework/

[6] Kim HY, Cho JS. Data governance framework for big data implementation with a case of Korea. In2017 IEEE International Congress on Big Data (BigData Congress) 2017 Jun 25 (pp. 384-391). IEEE.

[7] Brooks, Patti and Avera Health, "Standards and Interoperability in Healthcare Information Systems: Current Status, Problems, and Research Issues" (2010). MWAIS 2010 Proceedings. 18. http://aisel.aisnet.org/mwais2010/18

[8] Ruger JP. Shared health governance. Am J Bioeth. 2011 Jul;11(7):32-45. doi: 10.1080/15265161.2011.568577. PMID: 21745082; PMCID: PMC3988676.

The Role of Digital Health Policy and Leadership
K. Keshavjee and A. Khatami (Eds.)
© 2024 The Authors.
This article is published online with Open Access by IOS Press and distributed under the terms
of the Creative Commons Attribution Non-Commercial License 4.0 (CC BY-NC 4.0).
doi:10.3233/SHTI231311

Towards a Regulatory Framework for Workflow Improvement in Electronic Medical Records

Faiza ARSLAN[a], Jonathan MARCUS[b], Alireza KHATAMI[a,c], Aziz GUERGACHI[a,c,d]
and Karim KESHAVJEE[a,c,1]
a Institute of Health, Policy and Management, Dalla Lana School of Public Health,
University of Toronto, Toronto, ON, Canada
b Dr. Jonathan Marcus Medicine Professional Corp., Toronto, ON, Canada
c Department of Information Technology Management, Ted Rogers School of
Management, Toronto Metropolitan University, Toronto, ON, Canada
d Department of Mathematics and Statistics, York University, Toronto, ON, Canada
ORCiD ID: Alireza Khatami https://orcid.org/0000-0002-4175-5755, Karim Keshavjee
https://orcid.org/0000-0003-1317-7035

Abstract. Physicians have to complete several time-consuming and burnout-inducing tasks in their EMRs for everyday care of patients. Poor workflow design generates increased effort for physicians. In this study, we measure time doctors take to retrieve and review information in the patient chart at the beginning of a visit; one of approximately 12 tasks a doctor must do in the EMR during the visit. Information retrieval takes approximately 40 minutes per day. Automation could save 75% of that time. We estimate that if every family doctor in Canada could save 30 minutes through automation of just this one process, we could free up time equivalent to >3000 physicians and >5 million patients; enough to absorb the vast majority of patients who currently do not have a doctor. We know of no more powerful intervention than workflow automation in Canadian EMRs to increase the supply of doctors while simultaneously reducing a major cause of burnout. We recommend an accelerated research program to identify additional opportunities for workflow automation and a regulatory program to ensure that every physician has access to workflow automation in their EMR.

Keywords. Electronic medical records, workflow optimization, burnout, workflow automation, regulation

1. Introduction

The Canadian healthcare system is facing a pressing challenge, as approximately 50% of Canadians either don't have a doctor or are challenged to book an appointment with one, while an impending wave of retirements threatens to exacerbate the situation over the next five years [1,2]. Numerous factors contribute to this alarming trend, including physician burnout, time constraints, job dissatisfaction and cognitive overload. A significant factor is the burden imposed by Electronic Medical Records (EMR). Family

---

[1] Corresponding Author: Karim Keshavjee, karim.keshavjee@utoronto.ca

physicians spend twice as much time on EMR and deskwork as they do with their patients, impacting both efficiency and patient care [3]. Our healthcare system is unable to be proactive if we do not have an adequate supply of family physicians. The lack of primary care services is precisely why our system is so reactive and not proactive.

It is noteworthy that the principles underlying existing regulatory regimes for EMRs were developed in the 1990s and have not been re-evaluated in spite of the rapid advancements in technology over the last decade. Numerous tools have emerged to streamline processes and optimize workflows in other sectors, creating an opportunity to harness those advancements and adapt them for the benefit of family physicians and their patients. While some physicians have resorted to purchasing market-based solutions or employing medical scribes [3], these options are not universally accessible, affordable, or scalable. Additionally, some EMRs struggle to accommodate these assistive tools effectively, leaving many physicians at a disadvantage and leaving the healthcare system inefficiently resourced for primary care.

Addressing this pressing issue calls for the development of a new regulatory regime that incorporates advanced workflow features into EMR systems, providing advanced automation and ensuring equitable support for all family physicians

2. Methods

Observations of daily patient visits were conducted to capture the real-time workflow of family physicians. We measured the approximate time taken for each task physicians performed. To emphasize the time inefficiencies associated with repetitive tasks within the EMR system, we conducted a time measurement study focused on the retrieval and review of documents at the beginning of the patient visit. We categorized patients into broader diagnostic groups, including acute, chronic, and annual physicals. We carefully timed and recorded each task performed by physicians.

Additionally, we conducted semi-structured interviews with key stakeholders, including family physicians, patients, administrative staff, and the EMR vendor to gain insights into their perspectives on the workflow process.

Our project was based on healthcare process improvement and did not involve collection of any personally identifiable data; therefore, Research Ethics Board approval was not obtained.

3. Results

3.1. EMRs and interoperability create new work that did not exist before

We identified 3 stages of a clinical encounter that impact clinical workflows: pre-visit, visit and post-visit. The visit stage can be further broken down to retrieval, review and documentation of historical information, identification of opportunistic issues (e.g., disease prevention, medication renewal, etc.), obtain history, complete questionnaires, conduct physical examination, generate differential diagnosis, formulate diagnostic plan, educate patient, formulate treatment plan and formulate follow-up plan.

From the workflow assessment, we realized that compilation of the historical record can be extremely time consuming and is new work that did not exist 25 years ago. At the time EMRs were first being designed, data entry was the big challenge. Since EMRs had no historical information nor was interoperability widespread, reviewing information in EMRs was not considered to be a problem.

Physician regulators require them to document all information used in the course of providing care to patients, including information that may reside in different parts of the EMR; i.e., laboratory test results, diagnostic imaging reports, procedure reports, the updated medication list (from specialists, walk-in clinics and emergency department), treatment recommendations from specialists documented in consult notes, and so forth. Since all this information resides in different parts of the EMR, physicians need to retrieve the information, review it and document (henceforth 'compile') it before going onto the next step of providing care.

3.2. Retrieving, reviewing and documenting historical information is time-consuming

Table 1 shows the time it takes to compile historical information. On average it takes more than 1 minute to compile information for patients presenting with an acute self-limiting illness and close to 2 minutes for patients with a chronic condition or being seen for an annual physical examination. In a typical day where a physician sees approximately 30 patients per day, they may spend as much as 40 minutes just compiling information from the EMR! That is the equivalent of 4 patient visits foregone.

Table 1. Time taken to retrieve, review and document historical information (seconds).

Care Process	Acute Care Average (Range)	Chronic Care Average (Range)	Annual Physical Average (Range)
Retrieve and review	40 (20-60)	55 (20-90)	75 (30-120)
Document	34 (10-120)	61 (20-120)	44 (30-120)
Total time taken	74 (30-180)	116 (40-210)	119 (60-240)

3.3. Automating compilation of historical information could save significant time

We developed a logical algorithm for automation of retrieving and documenting historical information so that a physician could review it faster. We estimate that automation of this time-consuming compilation process could save 75% of the time currently taken in compiling information, since review is very rapid and efficient once all the data is in one place.

If we could save a physician 30 (0.75*40) minutes per day through automation of this one single EMR-related task, we estimate that each primary care physician in Canada could potentially be freed up for 2-3 additional patient visits per day, with a lot less cognitive effort. Multiplied by the number of primary care physicians across Canada (47337), this could open up an additional 95000 patient visits per day (the equivalent of over 3000 physicians); over the course of a year it would generate an additional 19 million visits (assuming 200 working days per year). The average patient visits their doctor 3.3 times per year, resulting in additional capacity for 5.7 million patients, addressing most of the current shortfall in primary care capacity in the country.

4. Discussion

Our study in a small clinic shows the promise of workflow automation in primary care. Even small efficiencies are greatly magnified when multiplied by the number of physicians across the country. Our study demonstrates that workflow automation is possible and that it cannot only save time, but can save cognitive effort, greatly reducing a key source of burnout when using an EMR. Even if our estimates are off by 50%, the small savings in time magnified by the number of physicians would lead to capacity to see an additional 2.8 million patients.

A key limitation of our study is that we only studied the first step in a multi-step process in one clinic. We recommend further research to identify workflow automation opportunities in 1) workflows in the pre-visit phase such as ensuring all tests and questionnaires are completed before the visit, 2) workflows in the in-visit phase such as documentation of the history and physical examination, formulation of the testing plan, the differential diagnosis, patient education, formulation of the treatment plan and follow-up plan, and 3) workflows in the post-visit phase, such as ensuring patients complete diagnostic testing, fill their prescriptions, attend specialist visits and providing appropriate support to patients to assist them in implementing the diagnostic and treatment plan.

5. Policy options and recommendation

Workflow automation is a very powerful tool that could have a significant impact on our healthcare system. Once improved workflows are developed and the software architectures are tested, a regulatory framework that incorporates these requirements into the EMR system would provide much-needed support to all family physicians. Replacing a family physician can cost between $250,000 to one million dollars and takes 6 years [3].We propose the following policy options for governments and key stakeholders to consider.

Option 1. Do nothing about workflow automation. Continue with the current approaches, which include funding additional teams, funding additional family medicine training spots and increasing funding for existing providers. The advantage of this approach is that investments have already been made, so let us wait to see what happens. There are many start-ups working in this area. Something is bound to work out. The disadvantage of doing nothing is that we lose out on a potentially high impact approach to improving physician supply that can deliver results in a shorter period of time than current approaches are capable of doing.

Option 2. Our recommended approach is to invest in research to identify more potential time-savings with workflow automation. If a small study can find such large time-savings, more research is likely to unearth additional opportunities for time-savings. The advantages of this option are that speeding up EMRs by improving their workflow capabilities can be put into motion very quickly and the benefits can be realized faster than it takes to train more family physicians. Results of the research can be shared with EMR vendors and start-ups who are already working to improve provider productivity, but without the benefit of a solid research program backing their efforts.

Option 3. To support market driven approaches already taking place by providing more grants to encourage greater uptake from the start-up community. This approach is likely to increase the number of solutions, but given the high costs of customer acquisition in the primary care space, it is likely to take a very long time and not lead to uniform adoption. Additionally, since research backing is missing from this option, it is unlikely to be sustainable or comprehensive, leaving many options unrealized.

There is another important reason for pursuing the approach we recommend. Primary care EMRs in Canada are a home-grown industry that does not depend on innovation arriving from the US. We cannot expect that the Americans, who have their own workflow optimization problems to solve that are completely different from those faced by Canadian physicians, will come to our rescue. Canadian EMRs are a uniquely Canadian problem that Canadians need to solve.

6. Conclusion

Our paper underscores the pressing issue of time-consuming, mind-numbing and repetitive tasks faced by family physicians during routine patient visits, contributing to burnout. Automating recurring processes in EMRs can save valuable time during patient visits and address an important source of health provider burnout.

To achieve this goal, we recommend a research program to identify more time-savings from workflow optimization and the software architectures that can deliver those workflow optimizations. Improving EMRs is likely to be much less expensive on a physician-equivalent basis and will generate the equivalent of thousands of physicians' worth of visits much faster.

By acting on and implementing the recommended changes, we believe we can alleviate the burden on our healthcare professionals, enhance patient care, and build a more proactive, sustainable and effective healthcare system for the future. It is time to recognize the importance of optimizing workflows and leveraging technology to create better working conditions for all healthcare providers in Canada by following a "Built by Canadians for Canadians" regulatory framework for EMRs.

References

[1]   Dangerfield K. "Half of Canadians Do Not Have a Doctor, or Battle for Appointments: Survey - National | Globalnews.ca." Global News. 17 Aug. 2023, https://globalnews.ca/news/9901922/canadians-family-doctor-shortage-cma-survey/#:~:text=More%20t han%20one%20in%20five Accessed 2 Sept. 2023.
[2]   More than 2.2 million Ontarians left without a family doctor: Family medicine news. Ontario College of Family Physicians (OCFP). OCFP News. 2023, February 9. https://www.ontariofamilyphysicians.ca/news-features/news/~287-More-Than-2-2-Million-Ontarians-L eft-Without-a-Family-Doctor Accessed 2 Sept. 2023.
[3]   Gardner RL, Cooper E, Haskell J, Harris DA, Poplau S, Kroth PJ, Linzer M. Physician stress and burnout: the impact of health information technology. J Am Med Inform Assoc. 2019 Feb 1;26(2):106-114. https://doi.org/10.1093/jamia/ocy145

The Role of Digital Health Policy and Leadership
K. Keshavjee and A. Khatami (Eds.)
© 2024 The Authors.
doi:10.3233/SHTI231312

Towards a Regulatory Framework for Electronic Medical Record Interoperability in Canada

Alireza KHATAMI [a,b,c], Jonathan MARCUS [d], Faiza ARSLAN [a], Aziz GUERGACHI [b]
and Karim KESHAVJEE [a,c,1]

[a] *Institute of Health, Policy and Management, Dalla Lana School of Public Health,*
University of Toronto, Toronto, ON, Canada
[b] *Department of Information Technology Management, Ted Rogers School of*
Management, Toronto Metropolitan University, Toronto, ON, Canada
[c] *InfoClin Inc. Toronto, ON, Canada*
[d] *Dr. Jonathan Marcus Medicine Professional Corp., Toronto, ON, Canada*
ORCiD ID: Alireza Khatami https://orcid.org/0000-0002-4175-5755, Karim Keshavjee
https://orcid.org/0000-0003-1317-7035

Abstract. All complex systems are potentially predisposed to failure. Healthcare systems are complex systems that are prone to many errors that can result in dire consequences for patients and healthcare providers. The healthcare system in Canada is under unprecedented strain due to shortages of healthcare providers, provider burnout, inefficient workflows, and a lack of appropriate digital infrastructure. We used failure mode and effects analysis (FMEA) to identify the failure modes for care provided in primary care settings. We identified failure modes in appointment scheduling, patient-provider communications, referrals, laboratory and diagnostic procedures, and medication prescriptions as the main failure modes. To mitigate the detected risks, we recommend solutions to 'close the loop' on failure modes to prevent patients from falling through the cracks, as vulnerable patients who cannot advocate for themselves are most likely to do so. We provide preliminary requirements for a regulatory regime for electronic health records that can reduce provider burnout, improve regulatory compliance, and improve system efficiency, all while improving patient safety, experience, and outcomes.

Keywords. Electronic health record, failure mode and effects analysis, healthcare system efficiency, interoperability, patient safety

1. Introduction

All systems have the potential for failure. In the case of the healthcare system, failures in primary care lead to downstream impacts such as increased healthcare utilization, healthcare provider burnout, failure to comply with regulatory requirements, and increased health system costs. To reduce errors, improve quality, reduce workload, and decrease costs, systems must become more proactive [1].

Healthcare systems are extremely complex because of the many interest holders (including patients/care providers, health care providers (HCP), payers, pharmaceutical

---

[1] Corresponding Author: Karim Keshavjee, karim.keshavjee@utoronto.ca

companies, health technology vendors, administrators, researchers, policy-makers and decision-makers), rapidly evolving knowledge and practice and the complexity of how care is delivered in a modern healthcare system [2]. Healthcare is delivered through a diverse group of facilities including but not limited to private clinics, hospitals, community health clinics, long-term care facilities, pharmacies, laboratories, radiology, and diagnostic imaging facilities. This diversity and a lack of coordination between them adds to the complexity of the healthcare system, which consequently increases the risk of errors in the system and reduces its safety and efficiency.

The Canadian healthcare system is under significant strain and is experiencing several serious problems including but not limited to a shortage of family physicians, registered nurses, and nurse practitioners; burnout of HCPs; rising and unmanageable costs; and an explosion in advanced health technologies [3]. In addition, the digitalization of healthcare in Canada has evolved slowly in comparison with other developed countries including the US, the UK, and Continental European countries [4].

An evolution of Electronic Medical Record (EMR) systems to encompass new interoperability features is required to tackle the complexity of day-to-day care of patients in our healthcare system. Introducing a "safety-first" regulatory regime for interoperability with EMRs in Canada could reduce the risks of patients falling through the cracks. Sound interoperability principles could improve patient access, optimize clinic and system efficiency by decreasing time spent on documentation and reviewing them; reduce inequity and patients falling through the cracks; enhance the simplicity of knowledge use and thereby reducing HCP burnout; and improve compliance with regulatory requirements.

Failure Modes and Effects Analysis (FMEA) is a reliability management tool that can proactively detect potential failures of a system and help identify promising methods to prevent them from occurring by assessing their causes and evaluating their effects. [5]. FMEA has been used extensively to identify and analyze the risk of failures in different fields of healthcare over the past decade [5, 6].

2.   Methods

We used the Institute of Healthcare Improvement's FMEA tool [5-7]. We focused on five main potential points of failure that frequently occur in the continuity of care based on our team's observations and documents from Canada Health Infoway, eHealth Ontario, the College of Physicians and Surgeons of Ontario, and the CommonWealth Fund healthcare performance indicators [3,7-9]. We performed a risk analysis on the causes and effects and obtained probability and severity rankings for them. We calculated the Risk Profile Number (RPN) for each failure mode. To calculate RPNs we estimated Occurrence (O) –the probability of failure of a process, Severity (S) –the severity of a failure, and Detection (D) –the probability of NOT detecting a failure. O, S, and D were measured on a scale of 1 to 10, and RPNs were calculated as O*S*D. RPNs range from 1 to 1000. Ethics approval was not sought. Our team of clinicians, health informaticians, and engineer-mathematicians brainstormed potential solutions for failure modes and effects.

3.   Results

We grouped identified requirements into the following categories: efficiency of clinical and administrative processes, regulatory compliance, patient safety, patient experience, data for operational effectiveness, ease of knowledge use, and last but not least equity. For example, for patient safety requirements, we identified laboratory tests not done, patient did not attend a referral, and prescriptions not filled. From the provider's lens, regulatory compliance and patient safety requirements could be viewed as an increased liability and reputational risk; e.g., license suspension or being sued.

Overall, we identified five high-level potential failure modes in an outpatient clinic: scheduling, communications, referrals, laboratory and diagnostic imaging testing, and prescriptions (Figure 1). We determined the causes and effects and assigned scores to O, S, and D according to our observations and literature search (Table 1).

Table 1. Selected FMEA analysis of an outpatient flow started with their intention to book an appointment to receive the proper care. Causes, effects, occurrence (O), severity(S), probability of not detecting the failure (D), and Risk Profile Numbers (RPNs).

Process	Cause(s)	Effect(s)	O	S	D	RPN
Scheduling	Phone busy, appointment too far in the future	Diagnostic delay, treatment delay	4	5	9	180
Communications	Message not sent, message not received, telephone tag	Diagnostic delay, treatment delay	3	5	10	150
Referrals	Message not sent, message not received, wrong specialist, specialist rejects referral	Diagnostic delay, treatment delay, downstream complications	3	8	10	240
Laboratory and diagnostic imaging testing	Patient does not complete, results lost in filing	Diagnostic delay, treatment delay, regulatory non-compliance	3	5	10	150
Prescriptions	Patient doesn't fill, patient doesn't pick up	Medication not taken, potential complications, increased system utilization	6	6	10	360

Table 1 demonstrates that the inability to detect patients falling through the cracks in key areas can lead to significant diagnostic and treatment delays, leading to worsened disease and increased health system utilization. Although not explicit in the table above, vulnerable patients are more likely to fall through the cracks, leading to worse outcomes for this subpopulation.

Siloed information limits the ability of HCPs to make the best clinical decisions, but unplanned interoperability could potentially increase the noise ratio significantly, adding to burnout and system inefficiency. We recommend that interoperability requirements focus on helping clinicians better detect when patients are falling through the cracks and follow up on them. Given that the number of 'defects' in the process is likely to be astronomically high, we also recommend that interoperability include robust risk profiling to ensure that those patients who are at the highest risk of complications and health system utilization are targeted first and that priority cases are no buried under an avalanche of missed visits, diagnostic testing, prescription abandonment, etc.

4. Discussion

An efficient booking and scheduling system is essential to facilitate timely patient access to physicians. A scheduling system that is interoperable with HCP EMRs could help detect the failure of appointment booking or referral completion, thereby preventing treatment delay.

A secure and robust communications system could enable clinics to identify when patients are not attending and provide appropriate follow-up. Since the risk of this happening is large, we recommend that clinics use this system with a risk profiling system to identify high-risk patients who need follow-up.

The process of ordering laboratory and diagnostic imaging testing is susceptible to the same potential errors. The College of Physicians and Surgeons of Ontario (CPSO) recommends that "physicians have an effective test results management system that enables them to effectively communicate test results to patients and take clinically appropriate actions" [11]. Clinicians need to decide on the importance of the results of diagnostic tests and procedures for the patient and decide on prioritizing communication. An interoperable EMR system with risk profiling can help clinicians track and follow up on high-risk laboratory results.

Medication prescription and dispensing is one of the processes that is frequently considered a failure mode in health systems [5]. The causes are diverse and can range from errors in prescription including drug interactions, not sending and delayed sending of the prescription and refill confirmations, wrong medication being given by the pharmacy, the patient not going to the pharmacy to get their drugs or delivery has not been arranged are just a few common causes. An interoperable EMR with risk profiling for high-risk patients (e.g., at-risk of developing kidney disease, blindness or stroke) could potentially help 'close the loop' on patients who fail to take their medications or who take too many because of prescriptions from multiple providers.

Despite improvements in implementing digital health solutions in Canada including the adoption of EMRs by more than 90% of physicians, these solutions and their functionalities could be used more efficiently [3]. Our proposed recommendations focus interoperability on improving quality of care, reducing cognitive workload, reducing administrative burden, improving system efficiency, reducing patient risk, improving compliance with regulations, and reducing health system utilization.

Limitations of our study include the narrow scope of the study for feasibility and reporting purposes. We focused on very simple but very common scenarios of encounter and care flow of a patient with their primary care physician, specialist, diagnostic laboratory and imaging facilities, and pharmacy. We only discuss the most common causes and significant effects in this paper. We also did not discuss technical aspects of interoperability.

5. Conclusions

We found several failure modes in outpatient care in the Canadian primary healthcare system that can and do result in significant effects such as increased risk to patients, HCP liability, and health system inefficiency and cost. Focused interoperability with EMRs can address most failure mode causes related to scheduling, communications, referrals, laboratory tests and diagnostic imaging procedures, and medication prescription and drug dispensing.

A regulatory regime for interoperable EMR needs the involvement of all interest holders and support from all three levels of government. This regime should encourage innovation and allow effective use of emerging technologies like artificial intelligence and machine learning.

References

[1]   Oas A. Failure Modes Effects Analysis - Taking The Final Workflow Step. Asset Management. Available from: https://reliabilityweb.com/articles/entry/failure_modes_effects_analysis_-_taking_the_final_workflow_step Accessed Aug 27, 2023.

[2]   Ortiz-Barrios MA, Herrera-Fontalvo Z, Rúa-Muñoz J, Ojeda-Gutiérrez S, De Felice F, Petrillo A. An integrated approach to evaluate the risk of adverse events in hospital sector: from theory to practice. Manag Decis. 2018;56(10):2187-2224. doi: 10.1108/MD-09-2017-0917.

[3]   Canada Health Infoway. Shared Pan-Canadian Interoperability Road Map. May 2023. Available from: https://www.infoway-inforoute.ca/en/component/edocman/6444-connecting-you-to-modern-health-care-shared-pan-canadian-interoperability-roadmap/view-document.Accessed Aug 27, 2023.

[4]   Canada: #17 in the 2020 World Index of Healthcare Innovation. Available from: https://freopp.org/canada-health-system-profile-17-in-the-world-index-of-healthcare-innovation-57d38eb31c58. Accessed Aug 27, 2023.

[5]   Liu HC, Zhang LJ, Ping YJ, Wang L. Failure mode and effects analysis for proactive healthcare risk evaluation: A systematic literature review. J Eval Clin Pract. 2020 Aug;26(4):1320-1337. doi: 10.1111/jep.13317.

[6]   Win KT, Phung H, Young L, Tran M, Alcock C, Hillman K. Electronic Health Record System Risk Assessment: A Case Study from the MINET. Health Inf Manag. 2004 Sep;33(2):43-48. doi: 10.1177/183335830403300205.

[7]   eHealth Ontario. EHR Interoperability Plan. Available from: https://ehealthontario.on.ca/files/public/support/Architecture/EHR_Interoperability_Plan.pdf. Accessed Aug 27, 2023.

[8]   College of Physicians and Surgeons of Ontario. Advice to the profession: Continuity of care. Available from: https://www.cpso.on.ca/Physicians/Policies-Guidance/Policies/Continuity-of-Care/Advice-to-the-Profession-Continuity-of-Care. Accessed Aug 27, 2023.

[9]   Schneider EC, Shah A, Doty MM, Tikannen R, Fields K, Williams II, RG. Mirror, Mirror 2021. Reflecting poorly: Health care in the U.S. comparing to other high-income countries. Commonwealth Fund, August 2021, 1-39.

[10]   Picard A. Survey says: Improve access to health care – now. The Globe and Mail. August 21, 2023. Available from: https://www.theglobeandmail.com/opinion/article-survey-says-improve-access-to-health-care-now/. Accessed Aug 27, 2023.

[11]   College of Physicians and Surgeons of Ontario.Managing Test Results. eDialogue. Available from: https://dialogue.cpso.on.ca/2021/03/managing-test-results/. Accessed Aug 27, 2023.

The Role of Digital Health Policy and Leadership
K. Keshavjee and A. Khatami (Eds.)
© *2024 The Authors.*
This article is published online with Open Access by IOS Press and distributed under the terms
of the Creative Commons Attribution Non-Commercial License 4.0 (CC BY-NC 4.0).
doi:10.3233/SHTI231313

Towards a Regulatory Framework for Electronic Medical Record Data Visualization

Rahul Shetty[a,1] and Karim Keshavjee[a,b]

[a] *InfoClin Inc, Toronto, ON, Canada*
[b] *Institute of Health Policy, Management and Evaluation, Dalla Lana School of Public Health, University of Toronto, Toronto, ON, Canada*
ORCiD ID: Karim Keshavjee https://orcid.org/0000-0003-1317-7035

Abstract. Physicians struggle to retrieve data from electronic medical records. We evaluated a digital tool that enhances physician efficiency in retrieving and analyzing patient information for treatment decision-making. Our use case is the care of diabetic patients. Evaluation results showed that healthcare providers who used the i4C (Insights for Care) dashboard experienced greater time efficiency than those who used traditional EMR information retrieval methods. A comprehensive evaluation of the i4C Dashboard confirms its effectiveness in facilitating diabetic care data management, as well as its potential application to a wide range of healthcare scenarios. In order to further maximize its effectiveness on clinical efficiency and patient care, future research should focus on improving its usability and scalability.

Keywords. Electronic medical records, diabetic care, user experience, time efficiency, digital health tools, quality improvement, primary care

1. Introduction

Efficient management of patient data is crucial for providing high-quality care. Electronic medical records (EMRs) have revolutionized the way healthcare providers collect, store and access patient information. However, navigating and retrieving data from EMRs is time-consuming and cumbersome for clinicians, which contributes to clinician burnout and hinders provider productivity [1,2].

Digital health dashboards aim to simplify clinicians' access to and analysis of patient data. This tool is designed to improve the efficiency of data retrieval from EMRs for treatment planning. Reviewing all relevant information before making treatment decisions is a critical step to prevent prescribing errors. In many cases, decision-making information is buried in a variety of data tables within the EMR, creating delays in and increasing the cognitive overhead of treatment planning. An intuitive and efficient dashboard can streamline data retrieval workflows and enable more effective real-time decision-making. The dashboard offers a technological solution that is not only more efficient but also potentially transformative for healthcare settings, particularly in the management of diabetes and other chronic diseases.

---

[1] Corresponding Author: Rahul Shetty, r.shetty@mail.utoronto.ca

2.   Methods

The primary purpose of the evaluation was to assess the relative efficiency of the i4C dashboard against Native Query in the EMR in clinical data retrieval within the context of diabetes care. We conducted a timed evaluation to study the efficiency of the i4C dashboard (*OntarioMD*) in the context of diabetes care. We compared clinicians' time spent on data retrieval using the i4C dashboard (i4C) compared with in-built EMR data retrieval methods (Native Query).

In a crossover evaluation design, 10 primary care physicians reviewed 10 elements of diabetes care data; the physicians used their own computer and EMR system. They were randomly allocated to initially use either i4C or Native Query and then switched to the other method. Two independent observers recorded the time taken to perform the tasks. Ethics approval was not required for this study because it was categorized as a co-design Quality Improvement study. The primary focus is on enhancing operational processes or systems rather than on patient outcomes or clinical interventions.

3.   Results

3.1. Clinicians save significant time when using a digital data retrieval tool

Clinicians using i4C dashboard saved significant time, outperforming themselves when using Native Query. Specifically, i4C users took a maximum of 33 seconds to find information from patients, compared to nearly 2250 seconds with Native Query. The mean time for i4c was 13 seconds compared to a mean time in Native Query of 315 seconds.

i4C dashboard also demonstrated more consistent performance, with a lower standard deviation in search times of 9.61 seconds compared to 628.30 seconds with Native Query, as shown in Figure 1.

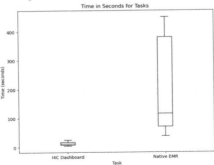

Figure 1. Comparison of the maximum time, mean time, and standard deviation in seconds between the i4C dashboard and native query.

3.2. Potential time saving with a dashboard tool

Table 1: Potential time saved by clinicians per day using dashboard.

Metric	Calculation	Result
Time saved per search	315 seconds (Native Query) – 13 seconds (i4C)	302 seconds
Total time saved per day per clinician	5 searches/day x 302 seconds/search	302 seconds/day (approx. 25.17minutes/day)
Additional patients that can be seen per clinician per day	25.17 minutes saved/day at 15 minutes per patient	Approx. 1.678 additional patients per day per clinician
Additional patients that could be seen across Canada per day	1.67 additional patients/doctor/day x 80,000 doctors across Canada	Approx. 134,240 additional patient visits/day
Physician Equivalents Freed Up	134,240 patients per day 1 doctor sees 30 patients/day	Equivalent of 4,474 additional doctors added to the system.

4. Discussion

The evaluation study demonstrates that the i4C Dashboard integrated to the EMR significantly reduces data retrieval time for care of individuals with diabetes by primary care physicians, halving the time compared to conventional methods and aligning with previous research on the efficiency benefits of integrated dashboards [3,4].

Qualitative analysis revealed positive feedback from clinicians regarding the user experience of the i4C dashboard. User-centered design principles should continue to be prioritized to optimize the usability and acceptance of such tools along with quality improvement [5,6].

As a result of the i4C Dashboard evaluation, it is essential to consider the implications of such efficient data retrieval tools across healthcare systems and strategize for their implementation. In the study, the dashboard was demonstrated to be a time-saving tool for diabetic care, and to improve user experience, suggesting the potential for bridging care gaps and reducing clinician burnout. Difficulties in EMR use not only affects the quality of care provided by clinicians but also leads to physician burnout and decreases the efficiency of the healthcare system as a whole when the inefficiencies are experienced by the large numbers of family physicians across Canada. The successful implementation of the dashboard provides evidence that data-driven tools can improve efficiency and reduce the burden of EMRs on healthcare professionals. With these advantages in mind, we examine various policy approaches for the widespread and rapid integration of these technologies, emphasizing their role in elevating healthcare quality and operational efficiency.

4.1. Policy options for rolling out data retrieval tools to enhance physician efficiency

We consider 3 policy options for rolling out physician efficiency enhancing tools for data visualization and for improving treatment formulation.

Option 1. Maintain the status quo, which is continuing with inefficient EMR systems that consume significant clinician time and contribute to burnout. The advantage of this option is that there are no expenditures to make and no risks of failed technology to explain. There is also no need to engage EMR vendors in a project that they are likely to resist because of the high costs and effort associated with change. This option does not address existing care gaps; provider burnout caused by poor EMR usability nor improve the quality of healthcare provided. It also does not address the shortage of family physicians in Canada.

Option 2. Allow market players to develop data retrieval tools and integrated dashboards and charge what the market will support. This approach is inefficient, slow to move ahead and will end up costing too much as the cost of customer acquisition in this space is too high. The benefits of the tools will not be achieved or will be achieved in a too long time framework.

Option 3. Design and develop a regulatory framework that ensures that every EMR embeds data retrieval and analytics tools into its system. This tool not only achieves significant time savings—freeing clinicians up to see thousands of additional patients each day—but also enhances the user experience and identifies care gaps more effectively. This makes it a cost-effective solution that can enhance healthcare quality and reduce clinician burnout, all in a single intervention.

Therefore, Option 3 could potentially save around 25 minutes per day per physician across Canada, freeing up substantial time for patient care. In summary, Option 3 offers a technological solution that is not only more efficient but also potentially transformative for healthcare settings, particularly in the management of patients with chronic diseases. The study delves into the dashboard's functionalities and algorithms, demonstrating its ability to provide clinicians with actionable insights for improved patient care in diabetes management [7,8]. Electronic medical records must be enhanced to increase efficiency and reduce time spent on administration. Hiring more doctors is the only alternative to technology tools. Our study suggests we would need to hire 4,000 more primary care physicians, a considerably more costly and time-consuming solution.

5. Conclusion

To comprehensively validate these promising findings, additional research with large, diverse clinician samples across different healthcare settings is required. Its limitations include a small sample size and a narrow focus. In the study, the EMR integrated dashboard was validated as an effective means of optimizing diabetes care data retrieval. This suggests its applicability to several healthcare specialties. Clinicians have reported significant time savings, which is indicative of the tool's potential for widespread use. The scalability, interoperability, and user-centric design of the system should be refined in future research to improve its impact on clinical practice and patient outcomes. OntarioMD and provincial governments could integrate such dashboard technology into future EMR development, saving them both time and money in the long run.

Acknowledgment

We would like to extend our gratitude to *OntarioMD* in Toronto, Canada, for their invaluable support and collaboration throughout the course of this project.

References

[1] Smith J, Brown A, Johnson K. Clinician burnout and the impact on healthcare outcomes. J Clin Psychol Med Settings. 2020; 27(2): 300–309. doi:10.1007/s10880-020-09677-8

[2] Johnson L, Williams M. The financial burden of clinician burnout. Health Aff. 2019; 38(11): 1842–1849. doi:10.1377/hlthaff.2019.01452

[3] Wilson D, Roberts E, Jones P. Evaluating the efficiency of EMR-integrated dashboards in reducing clinician burnout: A systematic literature review. Health Informatics J. 2019; 25(2): 98–114.

[4] Doe J, Smith R, Lee S. Efficiency of integrated dashboards in healthcare. J Med Syst. 2018; 42(8): 148. doi:10.1007/s10916-018-1003-4

[5] Brown S, Green A. Best practices for user-centered design in healthcare. J Biomed Inform. 2021; 114: 103709. doi: 10.1016/j.jbi.2021.103709

[6] White E, Smith L. Technology and quality improvement in healthcare. Qual Saf Health Care. 2019; 28(2): 139–145. doi:10.1136/qshc-2018-008472

[7] Canadian Institute for Health Information. Physician statistics in Canada, 2021 [Internet]. [cited 2023 Sep 12]. Available from: https://www.cihi.ca/en/physicians

[8] Canada Health info way. EMR Adoption among Primary Care Physicians, 2021 [Internet]. [cited 2023 Sep 12]. Available from: https://insights.infoway-inforoute.ca/cma-digital-health-use/

The Role of Digital Health Policy and Leadership
K. Keshavjee and A. Khatami (Eds.)
© 2024 The Authors.
This article is published online with Open Access by IOS Press and distributed under the terms
of the Creative Commons Attribution Non-Commercial License 4.0 (CC BY-NC 4.0).
doi:10.3233/SHTI231314

Lack of Data Access, but Not Availability, Hinders AI Training for High-Risk Conditions in Ontario

Fahreen WALIMOHAMED[a] and Karim KESHAVJEE[a,1]

[a] *Institute of Health Policy, Management and Evaluation, Dalla Lana School of Public Health, University of Toronto, Toronto, ON, Canada*

ORCiD ID: Karim Keshavjee https://orcid.org/0000-0003-1317-7035

Abstract. Advanced disease prediction is an important step toward achieving a proactive healthcare system. New technologies such as artificial intelligence are very promising in their ability to predict the onset of future disease much earlier than has been possible in the past. However, artificial intelligence requires training and training requires data. In this study, we report on the ready availability, but lack of accessibility and real-time access to healthcare data required to treat five high-cost diseases that are predictable using AI and preventable using well-established evidence-based therapies. There is urgent need for action on the part of governments and other interest holders to define and invest in the infrastructure required to make data for training and deploying AI at scale more accessible.

Keywords. Data availability, data accessibility, API, prediction, prevention. AI governance, artificial intelligence.

1. Introduction

Detecting disease early is a Holy Grail of any healthcare system [1]. The premise of early detection is making a predictive diagnosis and getting to treatment before the condition gets out of control and requires catastrophic care. As healthcare systems collect more data at various points of care, it becomes possible to predict disease much earlier than previously possible. The promise of early detection is the potential for reducing burden of disease, reducing health system utilization and extending life.

Artificial intelligence (AI) is rapidly becoming a mainstream technology with tremendous potential for providing not only early prediction of disease, but also to provide personalized recommendations to optimize the therapeutic dose of a medication or to provide recommendations for reversing the course of a chronic disease [2]. The benefits of AI algorithms compared to existing risk stratification models is their ability to classify patients into those at highest risk who deserve greater medical attention and their ability to re-classify those whose risk has decreased due to medical intervention.

Canada's healthcare system is characterized by fragmentation of care organizations, resulting in silos of data across the healthcare system. This makes it

---

[1] Corresponding Author, Karim Keshavjee, karim.keshavjee@utoronto.ca

difficult to train AI for chronic disease prediction and to train AI to assist patients in disease prevention, treatment, and avoiding hospitalization.

In this study, we investigate the gap in data availability and accessibility for training AI in a single jurisdiction (Ontario, Canada) for several important diseases that create a high burden of disease and drive significant health system utilization. We also propose recommendations for addressing the gap.

2. Methods

We identified and retrieved the costs of 5 chronic conditions that are predictable using AI, are preventable with existing evidence-based treatments, and drive significant health system utilization, using the Canadian Institute for Health Information's (CIHI) Patient-Cost Estimator [3]. For each condition, we conducted a goal-oriented requirements analysis to identify what data would be required to train an AI for the specific purpose of early identification of the condition and to assist patients to avoid the condition or exacerbation of the condition and subsequent health system utilization [4]. Finally, we identified whether that specific data is currently *available* anywhere in our healthcare system; whether it is *accessible* to researchers AND vendors of AI technologies; and whether it is accessible on a real-time or quasi-real-time basis through, for example, an application programming interface (API) for ongoing monitoring of AI performance and retraining of the AI as conditions change in response to interventions.

3. Results

The high-cost diseases we investigated are listed in Table 1. All are predictable using AI and all are preventable with known and efficacious medical interventions readily available and widely used in our healthcare system [5]. These five conditions alone account for almost three-quarters of a billion dollars of health system expenditure. Table 1 represents the costs incurred for 61,409 Ontarians who unnecessarily suffered a preventable disease [3]. Costs obtained from the CIHI Patient-Cost Estimator only account for direct costs of hospitalizations and physician costs during hospitalization. The Patient-Cost Estimator does not provide indirect costs (patient out-of-pocket costs, lost wages, etc.) nor does it provide other direct costs, such as for primary care, specialist care, diagnostic testing, and medications. The cost estimates shown are conservative figures and are likely to be much higher in actual practice.

Table 1. Predictable health conditions and their costs in Ontario (2019).

Condition/Disease/Procedure	Total Estimated Cost*
Coronary Artery Reperfusion	$357,245,528
COPD Exacerbation	$174,445,964
Stroke	$95,521,664
Acute Myocardial Infarction	$55,148,784
Lung Cancer	$32,341,147
Total	**$714,683,087**

*Total Cost = (Estimated average physician cost + Estimated average hospital cost) x Number of Patients

It would be misleading to state that all these cases are preventable, but addressing these diseases early would reduce a significant burden of disease for Ontarians and help reduce hallway medicine by a significant margin.

Data required for training of AI for the 5 conditions includes age, sex, height, weight, blood pressure, cholesterol, blood glucose, hemoglobin A1c, patient respiratory symptoms, smoking history, socio-economic status, air quality index and dates of outcome events such as hospitalizations, strokes, heart attacks and death. The data is routinely collected in a variety of care settings. The data required to predict these conditions are siloed in a variety of databases as shown in Table 2.

Table 2. Availability and Accessibility of Data for Training of AI in Ontario.

Data Source	Exists?	Accessible?	API?
EMR (Family Physician)	Yes	No	No
EMR (Hospital)	Yes	No	No
EMR (Specialist)	Yes	No	No
Vital Statistics (Birth and Death Registry)	Yes	No	No
Ontario Lab Information System (OLIS)	Yes	No	No
Pharmacy	Yes	No	No
Patient-Generated Data	No	No	No
Canadian Index of Multiple Deprivation	Yes	Yes	N/A
Public Health Ontario	Yes	No	No
Ontario Air Quality Index	Yes	Yes	Yes

● = Yes   ○ = No

Table 2 shows that most data needed to train AI already exists in Ontario, however, the vast majority of that data is not accessible to both researchers AND vendors, let alone accessible in real or quasi-real time through some form of API. Without adequate access to data, research on and training of AI cannot proceed.

4. Policy Options and Recommendations

Ontario has several policy options to make data accessible for training and deployment of AI for the prediction and prevention of significant diseases. The policy options below address important barriers that hinder accessibility, including privacy and security, lack of interoperability and the need to foster cooperation among players for long-term synergy while rewarding local innovation for near-term benefits.

Option 1. Status Quo: is to continue with the current approach which is to hope that the required AI will be provided by American vendors when they are mature and ready for the market. This is certainly an attractive option as it avoids uncertainty, the cost of investing in a speculative technology, and the risk of potential failure. The risk of pursuing the status quo is that when we finally do receive American AI, it ends up conflicting with Canadian values, goals, and socio-demographics because they are significantly different from American healthcare values, American market-driven healthcare goals, and American patterns of socio-economic distribution.

Option 2. Real-time API): our recommended option is to create the necessary policies and fund the development of key infrastructure that supports the development and training of home-grown AI. These policies could include a requirement that all health information custodians submit via real-time API a de-identified copy of their data holdings into a central data warehouse for the training of AI. The central repository would aim to house all data necessary for the prediction of diseases and would provide strict but transparent rules of engagement for researchers and AI vendors, with stiff penalties for breaches of the terms and conditions. Predictive AI could then be distributed to primary care providers for use in their EMRs to generate lists of patients at high risk of developing various outcomes. Prescriptive AI could generate personalized recommendations for the easiest pathway to reversing the trend of disease. The algorithms could be distributed by vendors with packaged advice on what evidence-based treatments the patient should receive to reverse the clinical course of their condition. Physicians could then provide those recommendation packages to patients, as appropriate. An additional benefit of this approach is that Ontario would become a leader in Canada for the development of community-based health AI and could be a supplier to the rest of Canada and potentially the world, since Canada's healthcare values are more in line with those of other socialized healthcare systems than America's are.

Option 3. Time-Delayed Batch: would be to empower Ontario Health or to commission third parties such as the Canadian Primary Care Sentinel Surveillance Network (CPCSSN), the Canadian Institute for Health Information (CIHI) or the Institute for Clinical and Evaluative Sciences (IC/ES) to develop AI algorithms using their *existing* data sets. These datasets are routinely extracted on a batch basis at periodic (quarterly to annual) intervals under strictly regulated conditions. AI algorithms would likely be updated on a less frequent basis than if an API were available but given the speed at which healthcare systems function and the speed at which diseases occur, the batch approach might be an acceptable compromise in the early days of launching an AI training program while these processes get off the ground. These organizations could work with deployment partners like *OntarioMD* and the eHealth Centre for Excellence to disseminate their algorithms to healthcare providers using existing dissemination channels. Without a profit motive, dissemination is likely to be slow and inefficient.

Option 4. Synthetic Data: is to use synthetic data derived from the characteristics of real data for model training. This option provides increased safety, but at the cost of model accuracy [6]. A lower model accuracy might be acceptable for research and publications, but would likely not be considered ethically acceptable given that even sharing identifiable data with vendors is considered acceptable and is routinely practiced in Canada under current privacy legislation. The question should be asked, why would we accept lower model accuracy when privacy legislation already contemplates this use and provides adequate safeguards for its use?

Our policy recommendation aligns directly with the Ontario Health Data Council Report: A Vision for Ontario's Health Data Ecosystem [7]. The integration, promotion, governance, and policies surrounding health data have been addressed in the recommendation to increase equity within patient populations. The collection of diverse datasets is important to prevent bias and would be addressed in our recommended option.

5. Discussion and Conclusion

This study documents the state of Ontario's ability to train locally developed artificial intelligence to achieve its own predictive and prescriptive infrastructure for important predictable and preventable diseases. Investments in IT infrastructure made over the last decade have led to significant growth in data assets. These data assets include primary care, specialist, and hospital EMRs and repositories for a variety of specialized data, including labs, digital imaging, and medications for seniors, welfare recipients and those on disability. However, many of those data assets now sit in silos, providing little value, other than being an audit trail for forensic and medico-legal purposes. Where data is available, it is only available for visual inspection and is not computable or usable for training AI.

Risks that must be managed in creating AI training infrastructure include 1) ensuring the collection of diverse datasets to mitigate potential biases in trained AI; 2) the dangers of misdiagnosis by AI in comparison to the current rate of misdiagnosis due to human error and finding ways for human and AI to work together to improve current rates of misdiagnosis; 3) de-skilling and automation complacency with AI can have dire consequences and is an area of active research in the informatics field.

We encourage Ontario and other jurisdictions to carefully consider how to mobilize healthcare data currently residing in silos to unleash the great potential for utilizing advanced AI technologies to improve the health of the population, decrease health system utilization, and increase capacity within our healthcare system. Even if jurisdictions would prefer to wait for other countries to provide them with AI models, they will need local data for fine-tuning the new models. Investment will be required, regardless of the approach taken.

Training of AI of course is not without its broader implications of having to invest in advanced data infrastructures, highly trained individuals, greater interoperability and robust information governance processes and procedures. However, many of these investments have already been made and now need to be harnessed. Organizations such as the Vector Institute, the Institute for Health Policy, Management and Evaluation, the Data Sciences Initiative, T-CAIREM and many others have significant expertise that can be leveraged for training AI. Deployment organizations such as OntarioMD and the eHealth Centre for Excellence can provide the necessary implementation support. Small incremental investments now could enable Ontario to become a world leader in the application of AI to proactive and preventive care. Investments in making necessary data accessible will enable the Province to leverage the investments it has already made in artificial intelligence to grow its healthcare software and AI industry and become a net exporter of health AI technology. Without the investments, Ontario stands to become a net importer of the technology, with the attend risks that that entails.

Our study is limited by the small number of conditions we studied, the Patient-Cost Estimator we used, and the rapidly evolving nature of data pipeline, data analytics, and artificial intelligence training. Further research could help identify additional savings and opportunities for training AI.

Acknowledgments

The authors wish to acknowledge Ryan Henderson, Daphne N. Kong, Archana Dhaka, and Muyideen Muhammed for their efforts in conducting the research for the results presented in Table 2, completed as an assignment in the Data Governance and Interoperability course at the Institute for Health Policy, Management and Evaluation.

References

[1]   Behr CM, Oude Wolcherink MJ, IJzerman MJ, Vliegenthart R, Koffijberg H. Population-Based Screening Using Low-Dose Chest Computed Tomography: A Systematic Review of Health Economic Evaluations. Pharmacoeconomics. 2023 Apr;41(4):395-411. doi: 10.1007/s40273-022-01238-3. Epub 2023 Jan 20. PMID: 36670332; PMCID: PMC10020316.

[2]   Kirk D, Catal C, Tekinerdogan B. Precision nutrition: A systematic literature review. Comput Biol Med. 2021 Jun;133:104365. doi: 10.1016/j.compbiomed.2021.104365. Epub 2021 Apr 7. PMID: 33866251.

[3]   Canadian Institute of Health Information. Patient Cost Estimator. 2019. Retrieved September 17, 2023, from https://www.cihi.ca/en/patient-cost-estimator

[4]   Nalchigar S, Yu E, Keshavjee K. Modeling machine learning requirements from three perspectives: a case report from the healthcare domain. Requirements Engineering. 2021 Jun;26:237-54.

[5]   Bauer UE, Briss PA, Goodman RA, Bowman BA. Prevention of chronic disease in the 21st century: elimination of the leading preventable causes of premature death and disability in the USA. The Lancet. 2014 Jul 5;384(9937):45-52.

[6]   Rankin D, Black M, Bond R, Wallace J, Mulvenna M, Epelde G. Reliability of supervised machine learning using synthetic data in health care: Model to preserve privacy for data sharing. JMIR medical informatics. 2020 Jul 20;8(7):e18910.

[7]   Ontario Health Data Council Report: A Vision for Ontario's Health Data Ecosystem | ontario.ca 2022. [cited 2023 Apr 25]. Available from: http://www.ontario.ca/page/ontario-health-data-council-report-vision-ontarios-health-data-ecosystem

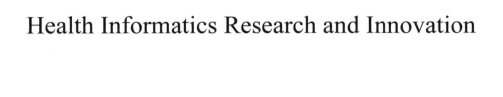

Health Informatics Research and Innovation

doi:10.3233/SHTI231316

Canada's Digital Health Workforce: The Role of Innovation, Research and Policy

Elizabeth M. BORYCKI[a,1], Claudia LAI[a] and Andre W. KUSHNIRUK[a]
[a] *School of Health Information Science, University of Victoria, Canada*
ORCiD ID: Elizabeth M. Borycki https://orcid.org/0000-0003-0928-8867
Claudia Lai https://orcid.org/0000-0003-3798-2880
Andre W. Kushniruk https://orcid.org/0000-0002-2557-9288

Abstract. The rapid growth of digital health and use of technology has led to an increased demand for qualified professionals in the areas of health informatics (HI) and health information management (HIM). This is reflected by the growth in the number of educational programs and graduates in these areas. However, to develop a culture of digital health innovation in Canada, the role of research needs to be critically examined. In this paper we discuss some of these issues around the relation between research and innovation, and the development of an innovation culture in health informatics, health information management and digital health in Canada. Recommendations for facilitating this development in terms of funding, granting and policy are also explored.

Keywords. Health informatics, health information management, digital health, education, research, innovation, policy

1. Introduction

The Canadian digital health market was valued at 16.88 billion dollars in 2022 and is expected to reach 66.07 billion CAD annually by 2030 (with an estimated growth rate of 18.6%) [1]. The digitization of healthcare in Canada has progressed at an exponential rate reaching 90% adoption of electronic medical records (EMRs) in physician and nurse practitioner offices and clinics [2,3]. The rate of hospital electronic health record (EHR) digitization is also significant with 81% of hospitals using radiology, laboratory and pharmacy systems [4]. Canadian consumers are no less interested in digital health technologies for health and wellness. Over 90% of Canadians use the Internet for health information [5], and 88% use mobile devices [6]. Alongside these changes, we have seen a significant growth in the number of health informatics (HI) and health information management (HIM) educational programs in Canada in response to workforce demands. Yet, despite this spending and general interest, many key stakeholders continue to suggest that Canada lacks a digital health innovation culture [7,8]. In this paper, we review the Canadian digital health innovation context (i.e., in terms of workforce, education and research), explore some of the gaps in the Canadian digital health innovation landscape, and provide policy recommendations to fill that gap.

---

[1] Corresponding Author: Elizabeth M Borycki, emb@uvic.ca

2. Background

2.1 Who are Canada's Digital Health Workforce?

Digital Health Canada defines HI as the professional discipline responsible for the modernization of healthcare through digitization. HI is the field of research, education and practice that involves the design, development, implementation and application of digital health technologies to support the use of health and healthcare data, information and knowledge. "HI enables and supports all aspects of safe, efficient and effective health services for Canadians (e.g., planning, research, development, organization, provision, evolution of services)" [9]. Digital Health Canada is a national organization that has been involved in developing HI competencies and certification [9,10]. Today, HI professionals work across Canada in varying roles such as HI analysts, clinical informatics specialists, data scientists, chief information officers and vice presidents of innovation. They form the human resource fabric of our digital health ecosystem and can be found in every sector: public sector (government and healthcare organizations), and private sector companies. HI professionals have extended their roles in healthcare to include developing, designing, and implementing medical devices, virtual care technologies, remote monitoring technologies, data analytics and artificial intelligent systems for health and wellness [10]. HIM professionals "transform data into valuable information", and "are responsible for the collection, protection, and accessibility of our health data." [11]. HI and HIM professionals have built Canada's digital health ecosystem.

2.2 HI and HIM Professional Workforce

The demand for HI and HIM professionals has grown significantly over the past few years with the increased digitization of our healthcare system and the shift towards virtual care. This digitization has changed the nature of health and wellness and how care is delivered. A recent workforce report identified a need for 39,000 additional HI and HIM professionals to effectively digitize healthcare. This number is estimated to be 48,360 HI and HIM professionals working in the field by 2022 based on an industry standard of an Annual Employment growth rate of 3%. When considered in the broader context of a health care workforce, HI and HIM professionals are the fourth largest discipline by number (Figure 1)[1], only surpassed in number by nurses, physicians and social workers. The HI and HIM workforce numbers are increasing, but when considered in the context of their roles in the design, development, implementation, and maintenance of digital health technologies used by all health professionals their size and contribution is consistent with the activities they perform across industry sectors.

2.3 HI and HIM Education: Universities and Colleges

Canada is a pioneer in HI education. It launched one of the first HI programs in North America over 40 years ago [12]. HI and HIM programs (n=34) now represent the third largest group of health professional academic programs by number (Figure 2)[1].

---

1. References for data for Figure 1 and Figure 2 can be obtained from E Borycki at emb@uvic.ca

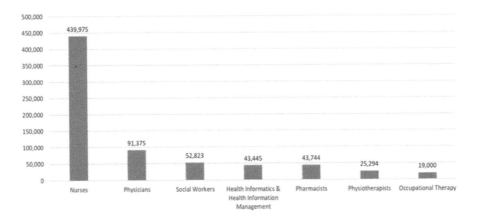

Figure 1. Number of health professionals by discipline employed in Canada.

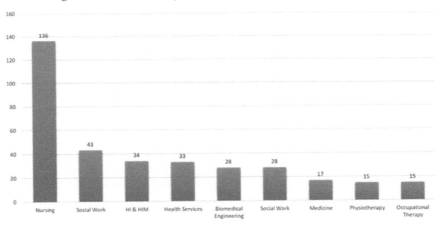

Figure 2. Number of HI and HIM schools and programs in Canada.

3. The Relation between Research and Innovation

Canada's growth in terms of HI and HIM workforce has been significant. This is consistent with the use of digital health technologies in every part of the healthcare system. Yet, creating a culture of digital health innovation remains a top concern for some stakeholders. Noseworthy and colleagues [13] argue for the need to create a learning health system that can advance technology and service innovations. A learning health system can only emerge when the "science, [health] informatics, incentives, and culture are aligned for continuous improvement and innovation, with best practices seamlessly embedded in the delivery process and new knowledge is captured as an integral by-product of the delivery experience"[14]. Provincial and territorial governments have invested heavily in HI and HIM programs in universities and colleges across Canada to meet the needs of our digital health ecosystem. However, there is a need to invest in HI and HIM research as well in order to close the loop in creating a culture of innovation (see Figure 3).

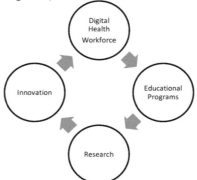

Figure 3. Digital health innovation in relation to research.

For HI and HIM professionals to develop a culture of innovation, there is a need to provide increased research opportunities to faculty and students specifically in the fields of HI and HIM. Research grants support innovation in university and college settings. Faculty funded research that takes place in universities or colleges leads to technological innovations and innovations in service design. By participating in research, students develop, test and pilot new technologies in academic settings, and after graduating implement innovations and create cultures of innovation within the organizations where they work. Such research investment creates a culture of innovation with faculty and trains students to become the future generation of industry innovators and leaders. To date, The Canadian Institutes of Health Research funds 12 Institutes. However, none of the Institutes is dedicated to supporting the critical work of HI and HIM faculty and students. This is despite technology having a ubiquitous role in supporting health and wellness for both the public and private sector. A dedicated research infrastructure is critical to advancing innovation in HI, HIM and healthcare.

4.   Recommendations for Creating a Culture of Digital Health Innovation

To build a learning health system with an innovative digital health force that can address the current and future demands of our health system, there is an urgent need to build a long-term research infrastructure that fosters a culture of digital health innovation in terms of health technology and technology service design. To address this issue, we suggest a number of policy recommendations:

- Create a new and separate Institute within the Canadian Institute of Health Research that focuses exclusively on funding HI and HIM research from academic institutions where HI and HIM programs are housed. These academic programs consist of faculty members who are internationally recognized for their HI and HIM research knowledge and expertise (and already train HI and HIM professionals in meeting Canada's workforce needs). Other countries have acknowledged this and brought this expertise into health granting for decades (e.g., National Library of Medicine, Agency for Healthcare Quality in the US).

- Provide funding to expand the number and capacity of HI and HIM educational programs to increase the number of highly qualified professionals, who have been involved in research and approaches to creating new digital health innovations.
- Increase funding to support continuing education for HI and HIM professionals already working in the field to build their knowledge base.
- Fund networks aimed at bringing together researchers from the 34 HI and HIM academic programs across the country to stimulate research and grow knowledge.
- Include HI and HIM as a discipline in the drop-down menus of submission systems of government and industry related institutes, programs and departments that fund research.
- Require greater collaboration among universities, industrial partners across Canada to receive funding, much like the EU funded research model for HI and HIM to enhance knowledge and innovation transfer.
- Increase the percentage of funding that is spent nationally on HI that would go into research on how to better design, implement and deploy digital health technologies.

HI and HIM professionals represent the 4th largest group of health professionals. The situation is much the same for HI and HIM educational programs. HI and HIM university and college academic programs are 3rd largest by number of programs (n=34) among the health professions. It is time to close the loop and create research infrastructure and opportunities for HI and HIM faculty researchers and students to create a digital health culture of innovation in Canada.

References

[1] Insights10. Canada digital health market analysis. 2023 https://www.insights10.com/report/canada-digital-health-market-analysis/ [accessed on 24-09-2023]

[2] Leger. 2021 National survey of Canadian physicians. https://www.infoway-inforoute.ca/en/component/edocman/3935-2021-national-survey-of-canadian-physicians/view-document?Itemid=103 [accessed on 24-09-2023]

[3] Borycki E, Sangster-Gormley E, Schreiber R, Swamy M, Feddema A, Griffith J. Electronic Record Adoption and Use among Nurse Practitioners in British Columbia. Can J Nurs Res. 2014 Mar;46(1):44-65. doi: 10.1177/084456211404600105.

[4] Gheorghiu, B., Hagens, S. Measuring interoperable EHR adoption and maturity: a Canadian example. BMC Med Inform Decis Mak 16, 8 (2016). https://doi.org/10.1186/s12911-016-0247-x

[5] Statistics Canada. Canadian Internet Use. https://www150.statcan.gc.ca/n1/daily-quotidien/191029/dq191029a-eng.htm [accessed on 24-09-2023]

[6] Canadian Radio-television and telecommunications commission. https://crtc.gc.ca/eng/publications/reports/policymonitoring/2018/cmr1.htm [accessed on 24-09-2023]

[7] Collier, R., Canada health care lacks culture of innovation. CMAJ September 10, 2018 190 (36) E1089-E1090; DOI: https://doi.org/10.1503/cmaj.109-5655

[8] Rigney G. Canada: #25 in the 2022 world index of healthcare innovation. https://freopp.org/canada-25-in-the-2022-world-index-of-healthcare-innovation-3db10d8d370b [accessed on 24-09-2023]

[9] Digital Health Canada. Health informatics professional core competencies. 2012.

[10] Digital Health Canada. Professional career matrix. 2019.

[11] Canadian Health Information Management Association. Health information overview. https://www.echima.ca/association/health-information-overview/

[12] Kushniruk A, Lau F, Borycki E, Protti D. The School of Health Information Science at the University of Victoria: towards an integrative model for health informatics education and research. Yearb Med Inform. 2006:159-65.

[13] [Noseworthy T. Innovation in the Canadian health system. Healthcare Management Forum. 2021;34(1):5-8. doi:10.1177/0840470420936709

[14] McGinnis JM, Aisner D, Olsen LO. The learning healthcare system. National Academies Press, 2007.

The Role of Digital Health Policy and Leadership
K. Keshavjee and A. Khatami (Eds.)
doi:10.3233/SHTI231317

AI Can Improve the Economics of Blindness Prevention in Canada

Swetha R. CHAKRAVARTHY[a,1], Dora MUGAMBI[a] and Karim KESHAVJEE[a]
[a] *Institute of Health, Policy and Management, Dalla Lana School of Public Health,*
University of Toronto, Toronto, ON, Canada
ORCiD ID: Swetha R Chakravarthy https://orcid.org/0000-0001-7046-7990,
Karim Keshavjee https://orcid.org/0000-0003-1317-7035

Abstract. Diabetic retinopathy is a leading cause of vision loss in Canada and creates significant economic and social burden on patients. Diabetic retinopathy is largely a preventable complication of diabetes mellitus. Yet, hundreds of thousands of Canadians continue to be at risk and thousands go on to develop vision loss and disability. Blindness has a significant impact on the Canadian economy, on families and the quality of life of affected individuals. This paper provides an economic analysis on two potential interventions for preventing blindness and concludes that use of AI to identify high-risk individuals could significantly decrease the costs of identifying, recalling, and screening patients at risk of vision loss, while achieving similar results as a full-fledged screening and recall program. We propose that minimal data interoperability between optometrists and family physicians combined with artificial intelligence to identify and screen those at highest risk of vision loss can lower the costs and increase the feasibility of screening and treating large numbers of patients at risk of going blind in Canada.

Keywords. Diabetic retinopathy, screening, artificial intelligence, risk prediction, vision loss, blindness

1. Introduction

Diabetic retinopathy (DR) is one of the most common complications of diabetes mellitus (DM) and is the leading cause of vision loss (VL) in Canada [1,2]. It causes blindness in the working age group, making it an important cause of disability, lost earnings, and lost productivity [1,3]. Its clinical costs are high as the symptoms are not evident until significant eye damage has already occurred. For example, glucose control and timely retina screening are key to minimize risk of severe DR and its associated VL. Apart from medical costs, a person with DR has non-medical costs such as loss of quality of life, cost of disability, lost productivity, increased insurance costs and lost earnings due to premature death/retirement, which is a major part of diabetes-related expenditures [3].

Ontario has the highest number of people with VL from DM (465,826 cases), followed by Quebec (283,935 cases) and British Columbia (166,754 cases) [3]. By 2040, DR associated VL is predicted to increase by 55% [3]. This will be a massive

---

[1] Corresponding author: Swetha R. Chakravarthy, swetha.ramanchakravarthy@mail.utoronto.ca

tragedy unless addressed early by regular screening, which can prevent 95% of the cases.

In Ontario, 440,000 patients with diabetes were not screened between 2016 and 2020 making 30% susceptible to DR in 3-5 years, and 50% may go blind in 5 years [3-5]. A recent study in Ontario revealed a continuing, accelerated decline in DR screening due to the pandemic, to as low as 20% in some populations which was influenced by their age group, ethnicity, and income [6,7]. The most vulnerable are at greatest risk.

There have been multiple attempts to solve the problem of not screening over the last 2 decades, with very little impact at the ground level for all the efforts and money spent on the problem [8]. All previous attempts used a customer relationship management system to reach out to patients at risk; however, scalability was a challenge as it is integrated neither with primary care, nor with optometry.

This paper reports on our economic analysis of two novel informatics scalable and affordable interventions to convert our system from the current reactive state to proactive.

2. Cost Effectiveness Analysis (CEA)

We used a CEA methodology for our study [9]. The population used is the 1.1 million people of Ontario who have DM Type 2, between 2016 and 2020. Forty percent, that is, 440,000 Ontarians did not undergo screening in this period [3].

2.1 Interventions evaluated

The informatics approaches we evaluated were 1) the Data Interoperability (DI) approach –interoperating data between optometrists and family physicians to identify those patients who have not received DR screening in the last year [10]. In this approach, every DM patient identified as not being screened for DR by a family physician, based on data received from optometrists on who has already been screened, is referred to an optometrist for screening. In Ontario for example, 440,000 patients would be referred. 2) The Risk Profiling (RP) approach –a modification of DI where only the 20% at highest risk of developing VL undergo screening by an optometrist. For example, in this model only 108,000 people would have to be recalled and screened instead of the full 440,000.

CEA was performed from the perspective of the Canadian Healthcare system and the perspective of a patient. Cost comparison was conducted in the following areas: a) the cost of inaction (the current costs), b) the cost of action (future clinical costs if implemented), c) the cost of the intervention (IT and management infrastructure to deliver the intervention) and d) patient out-of-pocket costs and loss of income.

The cost of inaction includes cost of treating DR with laser therapy and costs of VL for the unscreened population over a span of 4 years (2016-2020). The *cost of action* includes the costs of screening for DR (currently NOT incurred), laser treatment costs and blindness costs.

The cost of intervention is the cost of program implementation, including costs to identify patients at risk, data interoperability costs, the costs of recalling patients and the cost of human resources. For RP, it includes additional costs of designing, testing and validation of artificial intelligence (AI) or machine learning (ML) prediction models.

Patient costs include out of pocket costs incurred by patients due to vision loss. This includes direct healthcare costs and indirect costs due to the complications of blindness. It also includes financial cost of blindness, hospitalization costs, wellbeing cost, private expenditures on aids, equipment etc., rehabilitation cost, economic efficiency loss, medication cost and long-term disability cost [3].

Data values for each of the aspects of DI and RP approaches was based on costs obtained through literature review of existing studies done in Canada [3]. CEA and cost comparison of annual spending was conducted in each of the above-mentioned key areas.

3. Results

3.1. Cost comparison of DI vs RP

Table 1. Cost breakdown of Data Interoperability vs Risk Profiling Approaches.

	Data Interoperability	Risk Profiling
Percent impact	95%	90%
Cost of Inaction	$230 M	$230 M
Cost of Action (Additional Screening)	$56 M	$13.4 M
Cost of Intervention (IT infrastructure and Call Centre)	$90 M	$19 M
Total Cost of Program	$146 M	$32.4 M
Potential Cost Savings	$84 M	$197.6 M

Table 1 shows that the DI approach would prevent 95% of VL if implemented fully for 440,000 patients in Ontario vs. RP which would prevent approximately 90% of VL while screening only 108,000 patients. Implementation of DI would cost $146 million, while RP would cost only $32.4 million across Ontario. These costs are approximate average costs spent annually. Although RP costs are lower, it should be noted that it requires a new prediction model and research studies to confirm their effectiveness and therefore could take longer to implement. However, it is a significantly simpler solution for similar outcomes in the long run.

4. Option Evaluation

Results of this CEA strongly support the use case for improving DR screening strategies. There are three options available to address DR screening rates. Option one is to continue the current approach and do nothing. The benefits of this approach are that screening costs are not incurred and we avoid spending on IT interoperability, patient outreach infrastructure, clinician training and the costs of training and maintaining AI. However, this option is associated with rising healthcare costs due to rising rates of DR and VL.

The second option is to implement the DI approach to catch unscreened patients early. This approach is easier to implement and scalable. It requires sharing minimum data between optometrists and family physicians, making the transition easier. This approach is costly and would require significant investment in patient outreach and tracking infrastructure. More than 440,000 patients whom are not currently screened would incur additional costs of screening and time-consuming outreach plans.

The third option is to implement RP, the preferred and recommended approach. This approach identifies and screens only those who are at highest risk of VL. It requires fewer resources to maintain and is sustainable. Although it requires a longer time to implement, the total cost of RP will be less than DI and will be more feasible in the long term. Additional time is required to commission the development of prediction models whose accuracy relies on large, mixed data sets with minimal bias and are representative of the patients at risk.

5.   Discussion and Recommendation

Recently the Ontario Health Data Council published a report for responsible use of health data to establish a sustainable, learning health data ecosystem that benefits the people of Ontario [11]. This business case fits their vision and high-value system-level recommendations such as an integrated and accountable care approach between providers of different care settings, population health management identifying specific strata of our society, and the unique needs of individuals with DR. Both proposed approaches will focus on primary use of health data, not secondary use, with an objective of stratifying the population for targeted DR screening. This will entail data sharing agreements with essential policy requirements, process, and funding that facilitate sharing among all signatories with an entity commissioned to oversee it. Inputs from a report by Health Data Research Network Canada on *Social License for Uses of Health Data* could be utilized as a guide for next steps [12].

Risk prediction models have been used in clinical care for decades, and AI prediction models can enhance clinical decision making while fostering patient centered care. However, challenges like privacy, security and ethics need to be addressed for effective solutions to be accepted and trusted. Utilizing existing robust frameworks such as MINIMAR, TRIPOD-ML and PROBAST, can help address data transparency, minimal standards for reporting, potential biases and unintended consequences [13-15]. Further validation of the effectiveness of AI should be considered before implementing the policy recommendations.

Canadians witnessed a rapid digital health transformation in recent years with the COVID-19 pandemic. However, the increased digital uptake has only served to deepen the digital divide [16]. Fragmented systems, lack of data sharing and standardization have posed barriers to adoption. This could be overcome by prioritizing a data governance culture with clarity on data ownership, its accountability and IT infrastructure. Digital health interventions such as interoperability tools and risk prediction calculators can offer new possibilities for the early identification and treatment of DR, saving many Canadians from going blind.

References

[1]   Diabetes | the Canadian Association of Optometrists [Internet]. [cited 2023 Nov 13]. Available from: https://opto.ca/eye-health-library/diabetes

[2]   Diabetic Retinopathy | Diabetic Retinopathy NOW [Internet]. [cited 2023 Nov 13]. Available from: https://diabeticretinopathynow.com/diabetic-retinopathy/

[3]   Nguyen M. The cost of vision loss and blindness in Canada.

[4]   fb_canada. Diabetes: Cause of Working Age Blindness | Fighting Blindness Canada [Internet]. Fighting Blindness Canada (FBC). 2021 [cited 2023 Nov 13]. Available from: https://www.fightingblindness.ca/news/diabetes-leading-cause-of-working-age-blindness/

[5]   DiabetesCanadaWebsite [Internet]. [cited 2023 Nov 13]. Sight Loss Prevention and Diabetes. Available from: https://www.diabetes.ca/advocacy---policies/our-policy-positions/sight-loss-prevention-and-diabetes

[6]   Stanimirovic A, Francis T, Reed AC, Meerai S, Sutakovic O, Merritt R, et al. Impact of Intersecting Systems of Oppression on Diabetic Retinopathy Screening Among Those Who Identify as Women of Low Socioeconomic Status: Protocol for a Convergent Mixed Methods Study. JMIR Research Protocols [Internet]. 2021 Mar 5 [cited 2023 Nov 13];10(3):e23492. Available from: https://www.researchprotocols.org/2021/3/e23492

[7]   Impact of the COVID-19 Pandemic on Diabetes Screening and Incidence in Ontario | Department of Health and Society [Internet]. [cited 2023 Nov 13]. Available from: https://www.utsc.utoronto.ca/healthsociety/node/881

[8]   Tang C. Research Impact Canada. 2017 [cited 2023 Nov 13]. Watching Impact in the REF and How It Informs the Canadian Context / Le REF en observation : comment l'impact s'y manifeste, et son influence sur la situation canadienne. Available from: https://researchimpact.ca/archived/watching-impact-in-the-ref-and-how-it-informs-the-canadian-context-le-ref-en-observation-comment-limpact-sy-manifeste-et-son-influence-sur-la-situation-canadienne/

[9]   Guidelines for the Economic Evaluation of Health Technologies: Canada (4th Edition).

[10] Marcus J. Addressing a blind spot in care for patients living with diabetes - Healthy Debate [Internet]. 2023 [cited 2023 Nov 13]. Available from: https://healthydebate.ca/2023/02/topic/blind-spot-care-diabetes/, https://healthydebate.ca/2023/02/topic/blind-spot-care-diabetes/

[11] Ontario Health Data Council Report: A Vision for Ontario's Health Data Ecosystem | ontario.ca [Internet]. [cited 2023 Nov 13]. Available from: http://www.ontario.ca/page/ontario-health-data-council-report-vision-ontarios-health-data-ecosystem

[12] Burt J, Cumyn A, Dault R, Paprica PA, Blouin C, Carter P, et al. SOCIAL LICENCE FOR USES OF HEALTH DATA: A REPORT ON PUBLIC PERSPECTIVES.

[13] Hernandez-Boussard T, Bozkurt S, Ioannidis JPA, Shah NH. MINIMAR (MINimum Information for Medical AI Reporting): Developing reporting standards for artificial intelligence in health care. Journal of the American Medical Informatics Association [Internet]. 2020 Dec 9 [cited 2023 Nov 13];27(12):2011–5. Available from: https://doi.org/10.1093/jamia/ocaa088

[14] Collins GS, Reitsma JB, Altman DG, Moons KG. Transparent reporting of a multivariable prediction model for individual prognosis or diagnosis (TRIPOD): the TRIPOD Statement. BMC Medicine [Internet]. 2015 Jan 6 [cited 2023 Nov 13];13(1):1. Available from: https://doi.org/10.1186/s12916-014-0241-z

[15] Collins GS, Dhiman P, Navarro CLA, Ma J, Hooft L, Reitsma JB, et al. Protocol for development of a reporting guideline (TRIPOD-AI) and risk of bias tool (PROBAST-AI) for diagnostic and prognostic prediction model studies based on artificial intelligence. BMJ Open [Internet]. 2021 Jul 1 [cited 2023 Nov 13];11(7):e048008. Available from: https://bmjopen.bmj.com/content/11/7/e048008

[16] Superina S, Malik A, Moayedi Y, McGillion M, Ross HJ. Digital Health: The Promise and Peril. Canadian Journal of Cardiology [Internet]. 2022 Feb 1 [cited 2023 Nov 13];38(2):145–8. Available from: https://onlinecjc.ca/article/S0828-282X(21)00756-X/fulltext

The Role of Digital Health Policy and Leadership
K. Keshavjee and A. Khatami (Eds.)
© 2024 The Authors.
This article is published online with Open Access by IOS Press and distributed under the terms
of the Creative Commons Attribution Non-Commercial License 4.0 (CC BY-NC 4.0).
doi:10.3233/SHTI231318

Accelerating AI Innovation in Healthcare Through Mentorship

Divya KAMATH[a,b], Bemnet TEFERI[a,c], Rebecca CHAROW[a,b], Jane MATTSON[a], Jessica JARDINE[a], Tharshini JEYAKUMAR[a,b], Maram OMAR[a], Melody ZHANG[a], Jillian SCANDIFFIO[a], Mohammad SALHIA[b], Azra DHALLA[d] and David WILJER[a,b,c,1]

[a] University Health Network, Toronto, ON, Canada
[b] University of Toronto, Toronto, ON, Canada
[c] Michener Institute of Education at University Health Network, Toronto, ON, Canada
[d] Vector Institute, Toronto ON, Canada
ORCiD ID: David Wiljer https://orcid.org/0000-0002-2748-2658

Abstract. The adoption of Artificial Intelligence (AI) in the Canadian healthcare system falls behind that of other countries. Socio-technological considerations such as organizational readiness and a limited understanding of the technology are a few barriers impeding its adoption. To address this need, this study implemented a five-month AI mentorship program with the primary objective of developing participants' AI toolset. The analysis of our program's effectiveness resulted in recommendations for a successful mentorship and AI development and implementation program. 12 innovators and 11 experts from diverse backgrounds were formally matched and two symposiums were integrated into the program design. 8 interviewed participants revealed positive perceptions of the program underscoring its contribution to their professional development. Recommendations for future programs include: (1) obtaining organizational commitment for each participant; (2) incorporating structural supports throughout the program; and (3) adopting a team-based mentorship approach. The findings of this study offer a foundation rooted in evidence for the formulation of policies necessary to promote the integration of AI in Canada.

Keywords. Artificial intelligence, mentorship, best practice, health leadership

1. The missing piece to AI adoption- mentorship

Canada's adoption of Artificial Intelligence (AI) within the healthcare sector lags behind that of other nations [1]. Despite showing promising outcomes, its implementation encounters significant barriers related to organization and end-user readiness [2,3]. These barriers highlight the importance of taking a socio-technical approach that considers how technology, organizations, and end-user considerations need to be addressed to effectively guide AI implementation [2,3]. Recognizing this disparity, Healthcare Excellence Canada has provided recommendations to expedite the integration of AI in Canadian healthcare [4]. One strategy entails the development of mentorship programs

---

[1] Corresponding Author: David Wiljer, David.Wiljer@uhn.ca

that aim to facilitate skill enhancement and the exchange of expert knowledge [5,6]. Kang, et al. found that 60% of clinicians in a national-wide American study expressed interest in a mentorship program; however, only 65% of participants were aware of available mentors within their organizations [7,8]. These findings highlight the interest in mentorship opportunities by healthcare providers, along with the need for a program that connects those seeking guidance with experts in the field.

2. Program Overview

A mentorship program called the Innovation Hub was offered from August 2022 to January 2023, as part of a larger integrated knowledge translation project [9]. This program matched innovators and experts based on AI project objectives. Within five months, innovators developed a learning plan and connected with mentors for project guidance and experiential learning opportunities. To enable networking and community building, the program featured two symposiums and an online community platform for participants to ask questions and share ideas, resources, and project updates [10]. The program was designed using the CAMH health equity and inclusion framework to create an inclusive and safe learning environment for learners to express their opinions [11].

3. Analysis

The program successfully engaged 12 innovators across a diverse array of occupations, and experience levels. Most of the participants were healthcare providers and self-reported limited experience with AI development. Eleven experts were selected from diverse backgrounds including science, engineering, and ethics. Eight innovators and five experts participated in a post-evaluation interview to gain insight into the reach, effectiveness, adoption, implementation, and maintenance (RE-AIM) of the program [12]. This paper presents an overview of the effectiveness in terms of three domains: program design, AI project progress, and relationship quality.

3.1. Program Design

Despite having a positive experience in the program, there was a disconnection between the participants' initial expectations and their actual achievements. One innovator candidly remarked "[project] was just an unsuccessful idea, but I met some learning objectives. I mean it was a start of trying to develop something like this". Many innovators entered the program with the hope of completing an entire project from ideation to implementation within five months. These ambitious expectations of what the program and experts can provide led some to perceive their goals as unmet. However, all participants had successfully completed their project's initial phase: ideation. Simultaneously, experts struggled to define their roles, feeling incapable of guiding innovators through the entire project lifecycle and expressing lower engagement with program events. This led to fewer networking opportunities between experts and innovators that could be used for relationship building and knowledge exchange. However, all participants agreed that the structured components of the program, such as presentations, networking events, and one-on-one meetings, provided the greatest value for staying accountable and building knowledge. As one expert observed, *"That sort of guidance is really needed, because I felt like they were trying to bite off really big pieces of really challenging things to do in some respects without a good sense for what it would take to deliver."*

3.2. Project Progress

By program completion, all participants had successfully formulated viable project ideas and acquired a comprehensive understanding of the necessary steps for implementation. However, only a limited number of individuals managed to commence the development of their models. Several obstacles impeded the progress of these projects, primarily stemming from external resource limitations. For instance, many participants encountered challenges in accessing the required data for model development within their workplace. As one participant highlighted, *"where do I get the data from and who is the data kind of made available to... making sure again it meets all the privacy requirements."* Others lacked the necessary leadership support essential for project implementation. Some participants faced resistance from their departments and organizational ethics committees, which were not prepared to accommodate AI projects. One participant expressed frustration, stating, *"the ethics board doesn't really understand probably what I'm doing... they put another step for privacy... so, another sort of committee has to approve that. Honestly, I don't really get it. I just tried to challenge but they say no, you have to do it."* Lastly, a few participants lacked the technical expertise to code their models independently, necessitating external assistance that was not provided by the program. Despite these challenges, the mentorship program served as a motivating force and equipped innovators with the knowledge and networks needed to pursue their projects beyond the program's scope.

3.3. Relationship Quality

Interviews highlighted the importance of fostering strong mentorship and peer relationships through program design. The feedback concerning mentorship relationships was predominantly positive, yet highlighted areas for potential enhancement. Most participants found that even a few meetings with their experts offered invaluable insights into concept ideation, common AI implementation challenges to anticipate, and overall project feasibility. However, despite the value derived from these interactions, participants perceived some limitations in the mentorship matching process. Some participants felt that the mentorship lacked diverse perspectives, as one participant expressed, *"I got one good perspective from speaking to [expert], I felt like it may have been helpful to speak to a few more people."* Experts also acknowledged their limitations, particularly in guiding innovators with technical goals. One expert working in medical imaging and a leader of an AI program candidly admitted, *"I probably am misclassified as an expert...I think for anyone who comes in and has a technical goal, I'm not an ideal match."* To accommodate their lack of expertise, many put their mentees in contact with other experts from that domain.

Innovators consistently recognized the importance of acquiring knowledge through networking with peers, in addition to engaging with experts. Networking within the AI community proved equally advantageous as mentorship meetings. Innovators often felt isolated during the program and found inspiration and fresh ideas through interactions with fellow participants. That said, both experts and innovators emphasized the necessity of expanding the mentorship matching process to accommodate diverse needs. The formal matching process that was deployed ensured that clinicians lacking technical expertise receive appropriate support and have access to experts. However, many enjoyed the organic relationships that formed during networking events.

4. Recommendations

In order to facilitate the successful implementation of AI in healthcare and mentorship programs, we suggest the following three recommendations: (1) obtaining organizational commitment for each participant; (2) incorporating structural supports throughout the program; and (3) adopting a team-based mentorship approach [13].

It is essential to recognize that mentorship programs, while beneficial, cannot achieve meaningful change in isolation. Many departments lack an understanding of AI's potential to enhance operations and patient care, slowing down the implementation of AI within organizations [2,3]. To lay a strong foundation, organizational commitment should be part of any mentorship program to create an enabling environment for AI adoption. Organizational leadership must demonstrate dedication to innovation by sponsoring and supporting mentors and mentees. This commitment can take the form of an official contract outlining the organization's support throughout the project's lifecycle. Such support may include data access for model development, protected work hours for project development, and funding for project implementation. Additionally, other macro level changes such as organizational readiness and cultural shifts are integral for AI implementation. Without these systemic changes, the full value of mentorship programs may remain unrealized.

To help innovators leverage the program resources effectively, consistent structural support must be incorporated in the program design. A key design element includes setting realistic expectations for both mentors and mentees before the program's initiation. Organizational structures and support must be in place to ensure that innovators can make the most of mentorship programs as they are seeking support from the right stakeholders. Team-based mentorship may require different agreements between mentor and mentee tailored to their area of expertise and stage of development. For instance, the frequency of meetings and deliverables required for the development of an AI model may differ from what might be expected in the conceptual ideation phase. Additionally, given the variable timeframes of AI implementations, providing mentees with an AI implementation framework can help them structure their journey, stay on track, and break down a complex project into attainable sections.

In addition to organizational commitment and structural support, a team-based mentorship approach is required to support the interdisciplinary nature of AI projects [13]. As supported by the analysis of the relationship quality, a lot of learning occurred by engaging with people outside of the assigned mentorship pair. That said, a team-based approach can allow the mentee to be guided effectively through the various stages and complexities of an AI implementation project. This approach entails assembling expert teams with diverse backgrounds and skills, such as data science, computer science, diversity inclusion, and patient experience. The program's structure should be flexible enough to support a team-based approach, fostering increased collaboration and knowledge sharing among both participants and experts. Additionally, the program should avoid treating each team in isolation; instead, it should introduce additional sessions to facilitate peer learning, as networking was identified as a valuable aspect during program evaluations.

5. Conclusion

Mentorship programs provide an invaluable opportunity to bridge knowledge gaps and learn from experts. The Innovation Hub evaluation has identified several key findings and recommendations for future policies and strategies that are crucial for organizations seeking to embrace this transformative technology. With the right policies in place to inform design and delivery of educational programs, Canada could potentially emerge as a leader in AI education for healthcare professionals globally.

References

[1] Tran BX, Vu GT, Ha GH, Vuong QH, Ho MT, Vuong TT, La VP, Ho MT, Nghiem KC, Nguyen HL, Latkin CA. Global evolution of research in artificial intelligence in health and medicine: a bibliometric study. Journal of clinical medicine. 2019 Mar 14;8(3):360

[2] Choudhury A, Elkefi S. Acceptance, initial trust formation, and human biases in artificial intelligence: focus on clinicians. Frontiers in Digital Health, DOI. 2022 Aug;10.

[3] Sittig DF, Singh H. A new sociotechnical model for studying health information technology in complex adaptive healthcare systems. BMJ Quality & Safety. 2010 Oct 1;19(Suppl 3):i68-74.

[4] Healthcare Excellence Canada. Implementing Artificial Intelligence in Canadian Healthcare: A Kit for Getting Started. Ottawa: HEC; 2021 Nov.

[5] Köbis L, Mehner C. Ethical Questions Raised by AI-Supported Mentoring in Higher Education. Frontiers in Artificial Intelligence. 2021 Apr 30;4:624050

[6] Rahul Bagai, Vaishali Mane, "Designing an AI-Powered Mentorship Platform for Professional Development: Opportunities and Challenges," International Journal of Computer Trends and Technology, vol. 71, no. 4, pp. 108-114, 2023. Crossref, https://doi.org/10.14445/22312803/IJCTT-V71I4P114

[7] Kang SK, Rawson JV, Recht MP. Supporting imagers' VOICE: a national training program in comparative effectiveness research and big data analytics. Journal of the American College of Radiology. 2018 Oct 1;15(10):1451-4

[8] Kang SK, Lee CI, Pandharipande PV, Sanelli PC, Recht MP. Residents' introduction to comparative effectiveness research and big data analytics. J Am Coll Radiol 2017 Apr;14(4):534-536 [FREE Full text] [doi: 10.1016/j.jacr.2016.10.032] [Medline: 28139415]

[9] Wiljer D, Salhia M, Dolatabadi E, Dhalla A, Gillan C, Al-Mouaswas D, Jackson E, Waldorf J, Mattson J, Clare M, Lalani N. Accelerating the appropriate adoption of artificial intelligence in health care: protocol for a multistepped approach. JMIR Research Protocols. 2021 Oct 6;10(10):e30940.

[10] Accelerating the adoption of AI in health care [Internet]. Toronto: The Michener Institute of Education at University Health Network; 2021 [cited 2023 Sept 15]. Available from: https://michener.ca/acceleratingai/

[11] Agic B, Fruitman H, Maharaj A, Taylor J, Ashraf A, Henderson J, Ronda N, McKenzie K, Sockalingam S. Health Equity and Inclusion Framework for Education and Training.

[12] Kwan BM, McGinnes HL, Ory MG, Estabrooks PA, Waxmonsky JA, Glasgow RE. RE-AIM in the real world: use of the RE-AIM framework for program planning and evaluation in clinical and community settings. Frontiers in public health. 2019 Nov 22;7:345.

[13] Guise JM, Geller S, Regensteiner JG, Raymond N, Nagel J. Team mentoring for interdisciplinary team science: lessons from K12 scholars and directors. Academic medicine: journal of the Association of American Medical Colleges. 2017 Feb;92(2):214.

The Role of Digital Health Policy and Leadership
K. Keshavjee and A. Khatami (Eds.)
© 2024 The Authors.
doi:10.3233/SHTI231319

Improving Childhood Vaccination Rates with Process Innovation in Central Zone, Alberta

Sneha GURUNG[a,1]
[a] *University of Toronto, Institute of Health Policy, Management and Policy*
ORCiD ID: Sneha Gurung https://orcid.org/0009-0005-9320-2297

Abstract. This project aimed to accurately assess the current state of routine immunization program delivery in a Central Zone community in Alberta and provide actionable recommendations supported by literature review. Engaging with frontline public health nurses responsible for immunization program delivery in the community, contributing factors to low vaccination rates, process inefficiencies and policy gaps were identified. Based on additional literature, strategies to mitigate these gaps with the goal of increasing vaccination rates were proposed and validated. Although in this case, strategies to mitigate process inefficiencies were the most supported given program funding, a multi-pronged approach is still recommended to drive long-term improvements in vaccination rates.

Keywords. Vaccination, routine immunization, process, policy, Alberta

1. Introduction

Vaccination rates for vaccine-preventable diseases (VPDs) in Alberta for children are significantly lower than national target goals to prevent disease in this population effectively. For example, a 2019-2022 Alberta Health Services (AHS) report showed the immunization rate for the second dose of the MMR (measles, mumps, rubella) vaccine hovers at 74% in Alberta [1], where ideally 95% coverage is the national goal [2]. Immunization coverage refers to the proportion of a population that is appropriately immunized against a VPD at a point in time [3]. Figure 1 shows a steady national decline in the MMR vaccination rates, demonstrating that this is a growing problem faced across the country and based on a recent WHO report, across the world in the wake of the pandemic [4].

---

[1] Corresponding Author: Sneha Gurung, s.gurung@mail.utoronto.ca

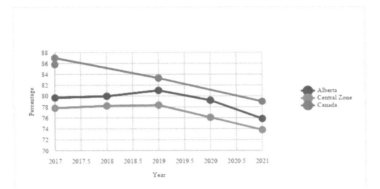

Figure 1. Percentage of children that received their second dose of the MMR vaccine by age 7, 2017-2021 in Central Zone, Alberta and Canada [1].

Alberta, unlike Ontario, has a single health entity called Alberta Health Services (2008) that was created in 2008. Alberta's Immunization Program operates under the authority of the *Public Health Act* and the Immunization Regulation, where the Chief Medical Officer of Health (CMOH) is responsible for monitoring Albertans health and providing recommendations to the Minister of Health and AHS [5]. The five zones of AHS (North, Central, South, Calgary, and Edmonton) operationalize the program with public health nurses being accountable for implementation, in accordance with provincial requirements [5].

This was an independent project with a focus on all routine vaccinations delivered to school-aged children in Central Zone, Alberta. The goal was to understand the current state of immunization program delivery and based on stakeholder engagement and literature review; develop actionable recommendations for the organization. Vaccines are well-known as being a cost-effective intervention, a study estimating a dose of the vaccine to cost approximately $20 in Canada [6], while delivery varies across local and provincial borders. Improving immunization program delivery can alleviate the downstream disease burden on our healthcare system and minimize public health costs related to the infectious disease response. One study analyzing the costs of public health response to the Ontario 2015 measles outbreak estimated total response to cost approximately $1.2 million, with almost half of the costs attributed to the local public health response to the outbreak.[6] This project's upstream approach to improve vaccination rates provides an opportunity to use public health resources effectively and proactively.

2. Methods

The first project objective was to understand why vaccination rates among school-aged children were falling below national goals prior to and now after the COVID-19 pandemic [1] in the Central Zone, one of the five zones in Alberta. As routine immunizations are delivered exclusively by nurses at public health centers, three AHS public health nurses (PHN) were engaged to understand this current state.

Conducting thorough research and validating the findings with frontline staff was key in effectively analyzing the problem in this project. Prior to engaging with these stakeholders, an initial review of Alberta's policies around vaccinations and a brief literature review to analyze the root cause of low vaccination rates in Alberta, was conducted. The findings were reviewed with the PHNs to validate that the understanding of the policy landscape was accurate. Preliminary findings from the literature was reviewed to narrow down the causes of low vaccination rates within this Central Zone city based on the nurses' experience working with the community. These nurses engaged were responsible for administering vaccinations for all age groups in this community, with PHN experience ranging from over 20 years to 6 years. They were first engaged through a focus group, where the causes of low vaccination rates and initial solution options were discussed.

The second phase of the project was to review their current workflows and processes to understand barriers and analyze strategies that could be implemented to improve processes based on the nurses' feedback, supported by evidence found in the literature. This was conducted via continuous email over the span of three months. The process used in this project are noted below and could be repeated in other organizations facing similar problems in vaccination rates.

3. Results

3.1. Understanding the Problem

In Alberta, routine childhood vaccinations are exclusively administered by public health nurses either in schools or at a community health center (CHC), with minor exceptions for COVID-19 and flu shots. There are currently no mandates in schools or other institutions (i.e., daycares) to ensure vaccination in children and adequate immunization coverage. From our review and validation, we realized that factors preventing timely vaccination varied across delivery zones in Alberta, but also across cities mere kilometers away from each other. For example, in this community, the nurses cited misinformation and mistrust in the government as one of the contributing factor preventing timely vaccinations while in a neighboring city, long wait times for appointments was cited as a common factor.

"Distance to the clinic wouldn't really be relevant in our situation, but in some other locations, for sure, like Red Deer – they always have longer wait times than we do." - PHN 1

"The resources are on the AHS website now, and I was thinking, well unfortunately, there seems to be a correlation with some vaccine hesitancy and skepticism with the government; the trust is not here. We say [to parents], go to this government website that says why we should vaccinate your kid, which is tricky if there's that mistrust there." - PHN 2

3.2. Identifying Processes

To further understand the current state and subsequently, design and validate solution approaches with the nurses, a basic understanding of the child/parent's experience was needed, in addition to the nurses' workflows. Two processes were developed that incorporated the child/parent, the nurses, and their IT systems by reviewing AHS website resources and interviewing the nurses. One was the process for vaccination within a community clinic and the second for vaccination within a school clinic. It was evident that in both processes, there was significant coordination and administrative work required by the nurses. For example, for school clinics, the nurses manually reviewed each child's vaccination history to determine the vaccines they were eligible for and were also responsible for coordinating clinic dates and consent forms with the school. Based on the nurses' responses, their typical workday consisted of these tasks along with vaccine administration at the clinics, with very little time left to engage with the parents.

The nurses noted that due to program decisions in recent years (before the pandemic), they no longer conducted in-person community outreach and education sessions and found this especially detrimental after the COVID-19 pandemic.

"We spent a lot of time doing that [classes on immunizations] and it's just in recent years that they haven't allowed us to do the post-natal [educational] classes and we really don't have time to do immunization sessions." - PHN 2

Current communication between parents and public health nurses now consists of newsletters, consent forms for in-school clinics and vaccination reminder phone calls, where parents may ask a few questions. The nurses believed that due to the government's actions during the pandemic and the reduced contact with public health nurses, they are now seeing more vaccine hesitant parents. This is evident in the parents' poor attitudes towards the nurses when they receive phone calls to remind them of overdue vaccinations for their child(ren) and nurses' experiencing an increased number of questions about vaccines from parents during the appointments.

3.3. Solution Design

With the information obtained about the current program delivery and challenges, recommendations were provided that would improve and streamline the current processes as well as compiling an initial list of strategies that were successful in other settings for their consideration. These were examined with the frontline nurses to validate what would be successful given the population they serve. For example, a technology solution implementation (online appointment booking) and process improvement in the current processes (utilizing existing digital reports) were validated, to redirect the nurses' focus on increasing outreach and education in the community. Some studies have shown that education is a factor in vaccination decisions and acceptance [7, 8]. Based on data from Statistics Canada, we found that approximately 18% of the population in this community did not have any certificate, diploma, or degree, and 30% have obtained a high school diploma [9]. So, increasing vaccine education in this population could likely begin to improve relationships between parents and the public health nurses within AHS's immunization program and potentially contribute to an increase in vaccination rates.

4.   Policy Implication

One of the strategies discussed with stakeholders was implementing a mandatory vaccination policy at public institutions like school, similar to Ontario's *Immunization of School Pupils Act*. The nurses had a mixed response, with some believing this is the only approach that will increase vaccination rates, while others believing that the strategy is too blunt and may cause more resistance and mistrust from the public. Comparison of two studies in the literature, one evaluating public attitude towards vaccines across over 60 countries and the other evaluating vaccine coverage after implementing strategies such as a mandatory policy did not demonstrate a causative effect on attitude post policy implementation. It seemed that countries with negative vaccine attitudes will more likely implement a mandatory vaccine policy [10, 11]. Another systemic review of mandates (mainly from the United States) found that generally, increase vaccination rates followed mandates [12]. For the project, further investigation is needed in Alberta to make an informed recommendation on using this policy lever, but initial stakeholder discussions suggest that mandating a vaccine policy may not as easily increase vaccination coverage.

5. Conclusion

Appropriate program and population evaluation is needed to identify challenges that may be unique to the local community to correctly determine a strategy to address low vaccination rates. This approach should be taken by organizations facing similar problems to deeply understand the problem and make evidence-based decisions. Looking past only using a technological solution to solve the problem and instead assessing all contributing factors (process, policy etc.) will likely yield valuable and actionable findings for an organization and contribute to improved vaccination rates.

References

[1] Alberta Health: Childhood Immunization Coverage Dashboard [Internet]. Government of Alberta [cited 2023 Oct 1]. Available from: https://healthanalytics.alberta.ca/SASVisualAnalytics/?reportUri=%2Freports%2Freports%2F310cb5ca-6959-4ccc-8c69-b63fbf765319&sectionIndex=0&sso_guest=true&reportViewOnly=true&reportContextBar=false&sas-welcome=false

[2] Vaccination Coverage Goals and Vaccine Preventable Disease Reduction Targets by 2025 [Internet]. Government of Canada; 2022 [updated 2022 Aug 16, cited 2023 Oct 1]. Available from: https://www.canada.ca/en/public-health/services/immunization-vaccine-priorities/national-immunization-strategy/vaccination-coverage-goals-vaccine-preventable-diseases-reduction-targets-2025.html#1.1.2

[3] Immunization Coverage [Internet]. Toronto: Public Health Ontario. [Updated 2023 Jan 25, cited 2023 Oct 1]. Available from https://www.publichealthontario.ca/en/Health-Topics/Immunization/Vaccine-Coverage#:~:text=Vaccine%20coverage%20refers%20to%20the,prevention%20and%20control%20of%20VPDs

[4] Nearly 40 million children are dangerously susceptible to growing measles threat [Internet]. World Health Organization: 2022 [cited 2023 Oct 1]. Available from: https://www.who.int/news/item/23-11-2022-nearly-40-million-children-are-dangerously-susceptible-to-growing-measles-threat

[5] Provincial Mandate: Alberta Immunization Policy [Internet]. Government of Alberta; 2019. [cited 2023 Oct 1]. Available from: https://open.alberta.ca/dataset/58d31634-61d9-469d-b95f-f714719b923e/resource/2a62de9d-4fda-4a9d-bd14-c81735943862/download/aip-introduction-provincial-mandate.pdf

[6] Ramsay LC, Crowcroft NS, Thomas S, Aruffo E, Teslya A, Heffernan JM, et al. Cost-effectiveness of measles control during elimination in Ontario, Canada, 2015. Euro Surveill. 2019 Mar;24(11):1800370. doi: 10.2807/1560-7917.ES.2019.24.11.1800370.

[7] Dubé E, Gagnon D, Ouakki M, Bettinger JA, Guay M, Halperin S, et al. Canadian Immunization Research Network. Understanding Vaccine Hesitancy in Canada: Results of a Consultation Study by the Canadian Immunization Research Network. PLoS One. 2016 Jun 3;11(6):e0156118. doi: 10.1371/journal.pone.0156118.

[8] Larson HJ, Jarrett C, Eckersberger E, Smith DM, Paterson P. Understanding vaccine hesitancy around vaccines and vaccination from a global perspective: a systematic review of published literature, 2007–2012. Vaccine. 2014 Apr 17;32(19):2150-9.

[9] Census Profile, 2021 Census of Population [Internet]. Statistics Canada: 2023 [cited 2023 Oct 1]. Available from: https://www12.statcan.gc.ca/census-recensement/2021/dp-

pd/prof/details/page.cfm?Lang=E&SearchText=Olds&DGUIDlist=2021A00054806034&GENDERlist
=1,2,3&STATISTIClist=1&HEADERlist=0

[10] Larson HJ, de Figueiredo A, Xiahong Z, Schulz WS, Verger P, Johnston IG, et al. The State of Vaccine Confidence 2016: Global Insights Through a 67-Country Survey. EBioMedicine. 2016 Oct;12:295-301. doi: 10.1016/j.ebiom.2016.08.042.

[11] Charrier L, Garlasco J, Thomas R, Gardois P, Bo M, Zotti CM. An Overview of Strategies to Improve Vaccination Compliance before and during the COVID-19 Pandemic. Int J Environ Res Public Health. 2022 Sep 3;19(17):11044. doi: 10.3390/ijerph191711044.

[12] Lee C, Robinson JL. Systematic review of the effect of immunization mandates on uptake of routine childhood immunizations. J Infect. 2016 Jun;72(6):659-666. doi: 10.1016/j.jinf.2016.04.002.

Patient-Focused Technologies

The Role of Digital Health Policy and Leadership
K. Keshavjee and A. Khatami (Eds.)

101

doi:10.3233/SHTI231321

Assessing Suicide Prevention Apps' Responsiveness to Help-Seeking Needs of Individuals Connected with Mental Health Services

Jessica KEMP[a,b,1], Hwayeon Danielle SHIN[a,b], Charlotte PAPE[a,b], Laura
BENNETT-POYNTER[c], Samantha GROVES[c], Karen LASCELLES[c] and Gillian
STRUDWICK[a,b]

[a] *Centre for Addiction and Mental Health, Toronto, Ontario, Canada*
[b] *Institute of Health Policy, Management, and Evaluation, University of Toronto, Toronto, Ontario, Canada*
[c] *Oxford Health NHS Foundation Trust, Oxford, United Kingdom*
ORCiD ID: Jessica Kemp http https://orcid.org/0000-0001-5159-4433, Hwayeon
Danielle Shin https://orcid.org/0000-0003-4037-4464, Charlotte Pape
https://orcid.org/0009-0007-8806-0778, Laura Bennett-Poynter
https://orcid.org/0009-0002-3741-7099, Samantha Groves
https://orcid.org/0000-0003-3271-7295, Karen Lascelles
https://orcid.org/0000-0002-6542-4379, Gillian Strudwick
https://orcid.org/0000-0002-1080-7372

Abstract. This paper maps suicide help-seeking needs identified in the literature, on to the features and functionalities of suicide prevention mobile apps using the adapted ecological model, thereby revealing existing gaps between help-seeking needs and available apps. This paper builds upon previous work by our team, which includes 1) a rapid scoping review aimed at identifying barriers and facilitators of help-seeking related to suicide within psychiatric populations, and 2) a review of suicide prevention apps, including a content analysis of app features and functionalities.

Keywords. Suicide, help-seeking, mobile health apps, digital health, mental health

1. Introduction

In Canada, there are 4,500 deaths by suicide per year, with suicide being the second leading cause of death among youth and young adults in the country [1]. Globally, suicide accounts for 700,000 deaths per year, revealing the immense burden of this public health priority [1].

Suicide attempts and self-harm significantly contribute to hospitalizations and other healthcare costs across Canada. The Centre for Addiction and Mental Health (CAMH) estimates that the economic cost of mental illness, including suicide and self-harm, in Canada is over $50 billion annually [2].

Corresponding Author: Jessica Kemp, jessica.kemp@camh.ca

The prevalence of suicide indicates a need for an improved understanding of the ways in which individuals experiencing suicidal ideation or behaviours seek help, and the existing barriers and facilitators that limit or support help-seeking in these populations. There is also a need to identify innovative solutions to support suicide prevention such as the use of mobile applications and other digital interventions, which have historically been used as an adjunct to treatment for depression, anxiety, and related disorders [3]. These considerations may contribute to reducing healthcare costs associated with suicide, help to prevent suicide-related deaths, and provide suitable mental health support that is responsive to individuals' help-seeking needs.

The purpose of this paper is to utilize the results of a rapid scoping review and mobile app store review to describe how previously identified barriers and facilitators of help-seeking relating to suicide for psychiatric populations compare to currently available suicide prevention apps. The gaps that are identified between individuals' needs and app features and functionalities will provide insights into what should be considered for future digital tools for suicide prevention including mobile apps.

2.   Methods

This study was conducted in three phases, building on a rapid scoping review and app store review conducted by the research team. The barriers and facilitators of help-seeking relating to suicide were identified in the literature, and the mobile app features and functionalities were then compared to the results to identify gaps.

2.1. Rapid Scoping Review

To determine the current state of help-seeking needs relating to suicide within psychiatric populations, a rapid scoping review was conducted using the Cochrane Rapid Review Methodology [4]. To narrow our search strategy, we focused on creating detailed eligibility criteria with the primary outcome being related to suicide, including ideation, attempts, and behaviour. Studies meeting this inclusion criteria were assessed for the reporting of barriers, facilitators, or needs relating to help-seeking to prevent suicide. Our search strategy was developed using keywords within our three concept domains (i.e., suicide, help-seeking, and psychiatric populations). The search was conducted during May of 2023 using the following databases: MEDLINE, Scopus, CINAHL, PsycInfo, and EMBASE. During data extraction, an adapted ecological model [5] was utilized to categorize the barriers and facilitators of help-seeking identified in each paper. This allowed for findings related to help-seeking to be grouped on five levels: individual, interpersonal, organizational/institutional, community, and national policy/law.

2.2. App Store Review

To identify mobile apps that are currently available to support suicide prevention, a search was conducted in the Apple and Android app stores using search terms related to suicide, suicide prevention, and safety planning. Apps meeting the following inclusion criteria were included: free to download, developed in the English language, and explicit provision of resources or tools to support suicide prevention. Eligible apps were downloaded, and data were extracted including descriptive information, security features, and personalization options. The availability of features and functionalities of each app was captured using the *Essential Features Framework* [6]. This framework assesses mobile apps for suicide prevention through 8 domains including general information regarding suicide, wellness, positivity and inspiration, distraction and alternate activities, safety planning, screening tools, helpful resources, and immediate help-seeking [6].

2.3. Mapping Barriers and Facilitators of Help-Seeking to Available App Features

Barriers and facilitators of help-seeking identified from the rapid scoping review were grouped based on the five levels of the adapted ecological model [5]. Features and functionalities of eligible suicide prevention apps were subsequently mapped onto the model if the app provided relevant resources or tools that addressed one of the mapped barriers or facilitators This process was conducted for all barriers and facilitators identified in the literature review and each app included from the app store review to determine which needs might be addressed via currently available suicide prevention apps.

3. Results

3.1. Rapid Scoping Review

The rapid scoping review yielded 42 studies from which barriers and facilitators were identified during data extraction. An overview of the number of barriers and facilitators identified is included in Table 1.

Table 1. Barriers and facilitators of help-seeking for suicide within psychiatric populations.

Ecological Level	Outcomes
Individual	27 studies reporting barriers, 16 studies reporting facilitators
Interpersonal	24 studies reporting barriers, 22 studies reporting facilitators
Organizational	26 studies reporting barriers, 15 studies reporting facilitators
Community	11 studies reporting barriers, 10 studies reporting facilitators
National/Policy	8 studies reporting barriers, 1 study reporting facilitators

3.2. App Store Review

The app store review resulted in the identification of 52 apps. Of these, 90.4% included general information about suicide (n=47), 21.2% included wellness resources (n=11), 63.5% included messages and information relating to positivity and inspiration (n=33), and 42.3% included distraction and alternative activities such as coping strategies (n=22). Safety planning features were included in 38.5% of the apps (n=20) and 17.3% included monitoring and screening tools to chart changes in mood, levels of distress, or personal suicide risk (n=9). The most common feature was information about helpful resources, such as contact details for suicide prevention helplines and local mental health services, which were included in all apps (n=52, 100%). Lastly, 90.4% of apps included resources for immediate help-seeking (e.g., direct crisis line) providing fast access through the app homepage (n=47).

3.3. Mapping Barriers and Facilitators of Help-Seeking to Available App Features

Facilitators and barriers of help-seeking across three levels of the adapted ecological model were addressed by features available in one or more of the 52 suicide prevention apps (Table 2). The most commonly addressed level was "individual", with 100% of apps (n=52) providing helpful resources responding to the facilitator of help-seeking for information about accessible support and self-help. Some apps also provided features or functionalities in alignment with help-seeking at the "interpersonal" level, with 11.5% (n=6) of apps responding to an interpersonal help-seeking need. At the "community" level, 94.2% (n=49) of apps responded to a facilitator of help-seeking. No app features or functionalities addressed barriers or facilitators at the organizational or policy level.

At the individual level, the app feature of signposting to helpful resources responds to the barrier identified in the literature review relating to help-seeking being impeded by a lack of knowledge about how and where to access support. In a fifth of cases (21.2%, n=11) this information was linked to location, supporting help-seeking at both individual and community levels. As identified in the literature review, capacity to cope has also been identified as a facilitator of help-seeking relating to suicide. Coping skills were addressed through a number of apps through positive and inspirational content as well as distraction activities and suggested coping strategies. A third facilitator of help-seeking at this level was self-awareness; this skill could be supported through the use of a number of the suicide prevention apps through the availability of screening tools (17.3%, n=9) or information about warning signs (82.7%, n=43), which could increase the users' awareness of their own mood, safety, and frequency of suicidal thoughts and/or behaviours.

The interpersonal level included the facilitator of emotional support and encouragement to seek help from friends, families, or other trusted individuals and was addressed by 9 apps. This was supported by providing the functionality for individuals to create and share suicide safety plans digitally with identified support persons. This feature allows friends and families to become more aware of an individual's level of vulnerability and needs and the ways in which they can provide support.

At the community level, the availability of resource information for mental health services and community-based care was reported as a facilitator of help-seeking. Nearly all apps provided content details of suicide prevention phone lines and emergency or mental health services available remotely or within the user's community to encourage help-seeking.

Table 2. Mapping of help-seeking needs addressed by existing suicide prevention apps.

Level	Help-Seeking Need	Essential Content Identified in App Review
Individual	Knowledge on where to seek help	52/52 (100%) helpful resources
		47/52 (90.4%) immediate support
	Capacity to cope	33/52 (63.5%) positivity and inspiration
		22/52 (42.3%) distraction/alternate activities
	Self-awareness	9/52 (17.3%) screening tools
		43/52 (82.7%) warning signs
Interpersonal	Support from family and friends	6/52 (11.5%) sharing safety plans
Community	Access to services in the community	49/52 (94.2%) remote and community-based services

4. Discussion

This mapping exercise identified gaps at the organizational and national/policy level as no apps responded to the facilitators or barriers of help-seeking associated with these levels. Though, this was expected as the barriers to help-seeking at these levels were often systemic issues that require complex interventions and national changes that cannot be meaningfully addressed through a digital means alone.

Barriers at the national/policy levels illustrated the impact of socio-demographic risk factors and the social determinants of suicide including health care coverage and cultural and societal values such as racism, gender discrimination, and perception of suicide [7]. Organizational-level barriers highlighted issues within healthcare systems, including dehumanization in mental healthcare, patients' distrust in healthcare, and the stigma associated with admissions involving individuals who have attempted suicide or have a mental illness. Although it is evident that these issues cannot be solved through the use of a digital tool, there are ways in which suicide prevention apps can momentarily relieve some of the impacts of these barriers and support clinical care. For example, the use of mobile health apps and other digital interventions have been shown to reduce stigma by allowing anonymity within supportive online communities [8]. Digital interventions that focus on building self-confidence and acceptance through peer support have been reported to be beneficial for individuals experiencing health challenges that are often highly stigmatized including HIV, eating disorders, and suicide [9]. These digital tools present a unique opportunity for individuals to seek help while reducing experiences of stigma, though they are not a replacement for clinical care. The greatest benefit is likely to be achieved through high-quality clinical care and the complementary use of suicide prevention apps that promote the use of safe and non-stigmatizing language.

In summary, our mapping exercise suggests that while suicide prevention apps can address individual, interpersonal, and community-level help-seeking needs, they have limited efficacy with regard to higher-level organizational and policy-related challenges due to systemic barriers such as socio-demographic factors, and healthcare system issues, including stigma and coverage. While we have discussed how apps can potentially reduce stigma and enhance anonymity, it's essential to emphasize that they cannot replace clinical care.

References

[1] Public Health Agency of Canada. Suicide in Canada: Key Statistics (infographic) [Internet]. 2022 [cited 2023 Sep 8]. Available from: https://www.canada.ca/en/public-health/services/publications/healthy-living/suicide-canada-key-statistics-infographic.html

[2] Mental Illness and Addiction: Facts and Statistics | CAMH [Internet]. [cited 2023 Sep 8]. Available from: https://www.camh.ca/en/driving-change/the-crisis-is-real/mental-health-statistics

[3] Shah A, Hussain-Shamsy N, Strudwick G, Sockalingam S, Nolan RP, Seto E. Digital Health Interventions for Depression and Anxiety Among People With Chronic Conditions: Scoping Review. Journal of Medical Internet Research. 2022 Sep 26;24(9):e38030.

[4] Garrity C, Gartlehner, G, Kamel, C, King, VJ, Nussbaumer-Streit, B, Stevens, A, et al. Cochrane Rapid Reviews Interim Guidance from the Cochrane Rapid Reviews Methods Group [Internet]. Cochrane; 2020 Mar. Available from: https://methods.cochrane.org/sites/methods.cochrane.org.rapidreviews/files/uploads/cochrane_rr_-_guidance-23mar2020-final.pdf

[5]   McLeroy KR, Bibeau D, Steckler A, Glanz K. An ecological perspective on health promotion program. Health Educ Q. 1988; 15(4):351-357.

[6]   Sequeira L, Kassam I, Kemp J, Wiljer D, Strauss J, Strudwick G. Mobile Apps for Suicide Prevention: Developing an Evidence-Based Framework for Essential Features. Poster session presented at: AMIA 2022 Annual Symposium; 2022 November 5-9; Washington, DC.

[7]   Pirkis J, Gunnell D, Hawton K, Hetrick S, Niederkrotenthaler T, Sinyor M, et al. A Public Health, Whole-of-Government Approach to National Suicide Prevention Strategies. Crisis. 2023 Mar;44(2):85–92.

[8]   Ali, K, Farrer L, Gulliver A, Griffiths KM. Online Peer-to-Peer Support for Young People With Mental Health Problems: A Systematic Review. Journal of Medical Internet Research. 2015 May 19;2(2):e19.

[9]   Flickinger TE, DeBolt C, Xie A, Kosmacki A, Grabowski M, Waldman AL, et al. Addressing Stigma Through a Virtual Community for People Living with HIV: A Mixed Methods Study of the PositiveLinks Mobile Health Intervention. AIDS Behav. 2018;22(10):3395–406.

The Role of Digital Health Policy and Leadership
K. Keshavjee and A. Khatami (Eds.)
© 2024 The Authors.
This article is published online with Open Access by IOS Press and distributed under the terms
of the Creative Commons Attribution Non-Commercial License 4.0 (CC BY-NC 4.0).
doi:10.3233/SHTI231322

Informing Mobile Health Policy for Pregnant Women in Rural Populations in Canada, with a Focus on Pre-Eclampsia

Shveta BHASKER[a*], Kadriye CANDAS[a*], Ashley GIRGIS[a*], Natasha
ROZARIO[a,1 *] and Praveena SANTHAKUMARAN[a*]

[a] *Institute of Health Policy, Management and Evaluation, Dalla Lana School of Public
Health, University of Toronto, Canada*

Abstract. Canadian healthcare suffers rural disparities, especially in maternal and
prenatal care. Drawing on a literature review, the paper highlights the potential of
mobile health (mHealth) applications to bridge this gap and improve maternal care
in rural communities. mHealth tools have great potential for knowledge and trust-
building among healthcare workers and pregnant women. To support the success of
these solutions, more funding and policy support are required. mHealth solutions
have a great potential for great economic savings while addressing healthcare
disparities and ensuring everyone has access to high quality care.

Keywords. Maternal health, pre-eclampsia, mobile health (mHealth), health policy,
rural communities

1. Introduction

Rural disparities in maternal and prenatal health are a significant source of concern in
Canada. Women residing in remote areas tend to have certain attributes that increase
their risk of poor pregnancy outcomes, such as comparatively high teen birth rates and
living in less prosperous communities [1]. Women in rural areas are 40% more likely to
suffer deliveries involving severe maternal morbidity and are 17% more likely to be
readmitted to the hospital when compared to their urban counterparts [1]. In addition, the
infant mortality rate is 2.6 times higher for those living in less resource abundant areas
[2]. Fortunately, mobile health (mHealth) has been acknowledged, on a global and
national level, for its vital role in rejuvenating healthcare [3]. Thus, this paper issues a
call to action for provincial health authorities to utilize clinician-facing mHealth for the
early detection of pre-eclampsia (PE), a potentially fatal complication of pregnancy
hypertension. The outcomes of mHealth studied in this scope of research, like PIERS on
the Move (POM), demonstrate that there is an immense opportunity for mHealth to
intervene to bridge rural disparities [4-6]. Ultimately, this paper aims to address rural
disparities in Canada by promoting policy-driven mHealth solutions focused on maternal
and prenatal care.

---

[1] Corresponding author, mail@natasharozario.com
* Equal contribution

2.   Methods

Academic databases including PubMed, Embase, and Web of Science were used to retrieve 18 articles for the rapid review with the following search sentence: "(((mHealth) AND (women)) AND (preeclampsia)) AND (rural)". The Covidence software program was used to manage the articles and 5 duplicates were removed. The inclusion criteria were pregnant women, children, mHealth diagnosis, management of pre-eclampsia, management of maternal health, health equity, health policy, and rural health. The exclusion criteria were non-pregnant women and any other digital health tool (telemedicine). The resulting 11 articles were screened as part of the title and abstract screening. 5 articles were examined in the full-text review to derive insights for the results table.

3.   Results

Table 1. Review of studies focused on maternal health mHealth applications captured in the search strategy, compiling study source, location, application name, and the most relevant outcomes.

Study Source	Location	mHealth	Relevant Outcomes	Intervention Barriers
Boene et al., 2021	Rural Mozambique	PIERS on the Move (POM)	Increased knowledge on pregnancy complications. Confidence in recognizing danger signs related to PE and administering injections for seizures. Accuracy measuring blood pressure.	Incomplete visits due to poor connection to pulse oximeter or battery life depletion.
Charanthi-math et al., 2021	Rural India	POM	Confidence in recognizing signs of labor. Comfortability accompanying pregnant women that require medical attention.	Incomplete visits and battery life depletion. Too many fields or complex to correct mistakes.
Kinshella et al., 2021	Rural Pakistan	POM	Earlier detection of PE and more timely decision-making to seek care. More effective and valuable delivery of community health services.	Patient concerns with data-sharing of photos.
Abejirind-e et al., 2018	Rural Ghana	Bliss4Mi dwives (B4M)	Improved knowledge and skills of health workers. Increased patient trust in diagnostic advice and motivated referral compliance.	Lack of education on intervention and patient distrust in B4M.
Wirth et al., 2018	Rural Bangladesh	uChek©	Processed 10-20 urinalysis tests within half an hour compared to standard of 1 test per half an hour. Reduced wait times and human error.	Barriers were not discussed.

Note. All mHealth applications listed target community health workers by assessing the risk of pre-eclampsia. B4M also screens for gestational diabetes and anemia.

4.   Discussion

The literature underscores the potential of mHealth applications as valuable tools for midwives globally, particularly in non-invasive screening for pregnancy-related complications such as PE, gestational diabetes, and anemia [4-8]. For instance, the POM app has shown significant effectiveness in predicting adverse outcomes of PE in rural areas of India, Mozambique, and Pakistan, improving maternal health outcomes, and reducing hospital readmissions [4-6]. Tailoring digital health interventions, like POM, for rural areas in Canada could benefit both patients and healthcare providers. This can alleviate the substantial economic burden associated with managing PE, which currently costs the Canadian healthcare system $8.6 million [9, 10]. Implementing mHealth apps holds the potential to save over $1.3 million in healthcare costs, despite the need for addressing challenges related to implementation and usability, offering a promising means for empowering midwives, and providing essential guidance and support to pregnant women in resource-limited settings [9, 10].

Ultimately, the value of mHealth's ability to promote knowledge and trust building will reap in higher quality care, proactive decision-making before adverse events occur, patient compliance, and patient empowerment.

4.1. Policy Options

Dubbed "a country of perpetual projects", it is rare for projects in Canada to move beyond the pilot stage to sustainable programs [11]. This is a waste of investment, research effort, and time, where there is a great potential to deliver better quality and access to care. To increase usage of mHealth tools to address PE, evidence-based apps with proven efficacy should be added as a service to the Schedule of Benefits. Having clear insurance coverage for these tools helps to establish long-term support for their usage and supports the sustainability of their implementation.

To help guide clinicians to effectively use mHealth solutions and integrate the tools with their practice, specific clinical guidelines are required. The Canadian Medical Association developed a few guiding principles for physicians recommending mHealth apps to patients but there are no explicit guidelines for how to manage and control data flow, interpret analysis or recommendations given by the app, or remain compliant with privacy regulations [12]. Clinical guidelines created by the Society of Obstetricians and Gynecologists of Canada for using mHealth tools to treat PE not only ensures a standard quality of care with the way these tools are used in clinical practice, but it also makes it easier to evaluate the success of these tools.

Because of the digital divide, rural communities tend to have less digital literacy skills, affecting patients' and providers' ability to use mHealth tools. To address this, Canada's Digital Literacy Exchange Program should be adapted to train patients and providers in rural communities to use mHealth tools with high fidelity. Higher digital literacy not only enables individuals to gain the full benefits of the tool, but it also helps foster trust in the technology and improves patient engagement [13].

In developing mHealth solutions as a tool to improve outcomes and access to healthcare amongst rural populations, it is also vital to make sure that these tools do not inadvertently become barriers for the very populations trying to be served. Infrastructure such as good network connectivity are integral to the feasibility of mHealth. However, with 38% of rural households lacking access to a sufficient internet connection, this is not a universally accessible resource [14]. One possible solution is to provide direct-to-consumer subsidies for broadband access for these populations. The government of Canada launched a similar initiative, Connected Families, in 2017 for low-income families [15]. Extending this initiative to increase access to quality healthcare to rural communities would be in keeping with Canada's Connectivity Strategy, which aims to increase access to stable high-speed internet to support Canada's social and economic development [16].

5.   Conclusion

A view of the healthcare system through a lens of rural health shows the inequities faced by rural communities. However, other sectors of healthcare also have underlying inequities rooted in racism, sexism, classism, and other forms of discrimination. While many discriminated groups have a unique history with the healthcare system and require their own individualized strategies and approaches, many can benefit from the same policies recommended in this paper. In continuing this work, more research is required on experiences and outcomes of discriminated populations, especially with consideration to intersectional identities. However, these disparities are ultimately systemic and while technology like mHealth tools can make a positive impact on the experiences of affected people, they do not replace policy interventions targeting the upstream social determinants and reducing the root disparities.

Acknowledgement

Thank you to Dr. Karim Keshavjee and Dr. Alireza Khatami for their guidance.

References

[1] Hospital Births in Canada: A Focus on Women Living in Rural and Remote Areas [Internet]. Canadian Institute for Health Information; 2013. Available from https://publications.gc.ca/collections/collection_2013/icis-cihi/H118-89-2013-eng.pdf

[2] Infographic: Inequalities in infant mortality in Canada [Internet]. Public Health Agency of Canada; 2019. Available from https://www.canada.ca/en/public-health/services/publications/science-research-data/inequalities-infant-mortality-infographic.html

[3] Notice: Health Canada's Approach to Digital Health Technologies [Internet]. (2018). Health Canada; 2018. Available from https://www.canada.ca/en/health-canada/services/drugs-health-products/medical-devices/activities/announcements/notice-digital-health-technologies.html

[4] Boene H, Valá A, Kinshella ML, La M, Sharma S, Vidler M, et al. Implementation of the PIERS on the move mHealth application from the perspective of community health workers and nurses in rural Mozambique. Frontiers in Global Women's Health. 2021 May 3;2:659582.

[5] Charanthimath U, Katageri G, Kinshella ML, Mallapur A, Goudar S, Ramadurg U, et al. Community health worker evaluation of implementing an mHealth application to support maternal health care in rural India. Frontiers in Global Women's Health. 2021 Sep 1;2:645690.

[6] Kinshella ML, Sheikh S, Bawani S, La M, Sharma S, Vidler M, et al.. "Now You Have Become Doctors": Lady Health Workers' Experiences Implementing an mHealth Application in Rural Pakistan. Frontiers in Global Women's Health. 2021 May 14;2:645705.

[7] Abejirinde IO, Douwes R, Bardají A, Abugnaba-Abanga R, Zweekhorst M, van Roosmalen J, De Brouwere V. Pregnant women's experiences with an integrated diagnostic and decision support device for antenatal care in Ghana. BMC Pregnancy and Childbirth. 2018 Dec;18(1):1-1.

[8] Wirth M, Biswas N, Ahmad S, Nayak HS, Pugh A, Gupta T, Mahmood I. A prospective observational pilot study to test the feasibility of a smartphone enabled uChek© urinalysis device to detect biomarkers in urine indicative of preeclampsia/eclampsia. Health and Technology. 2019 Jan 24;9(1):31-6.

[9] Liu A, Wen SW, Bottomley J, Walker MC, Smith G. Utilization of health care services of pregnant women complicated by preeclampsia in Ontario. Hypertension in Pregnancy. 2009;28(1):76–84. doi:10.1080/10641950802366252

[10] Mobile Health app development costs $425,000 on average, likely continuing to rise [Internet]. 2018. Available from: https://www.mobihealthnews.com/content/mobile-health-app-development-costs-425000-average-likely-continuing-rise

[11] Bégin M, Eggertson L, Macdonald N. A country of perpetual pilot projects. Canadian Medical Association Journal [Internet]. 2009 June 9. doi: 10.1503/cmaj.

[12] Guiding Principles for Physicians Recommending Mobile Health Applications to Patients [Internet]. Canadian Medical Association; [updated 2018 Nov]. Available from https://www.cma.ca/sites/default/files/2018-11/cma_policy_guiding_principles_for_physicians_recommending_mobile_health_applications_to_patients_pd1-e.pdf

[13] Martin T. Assessing mhealth: Opportunities and barriers to patient engagement. Journal of Health Care for the Poor and Underserved. 2012;23(3):935–41. doi:10.1353/hpu.2012.0087

[14] CRTC to improve access to Internet and mobile services across Canada [Internet]. CRTC Canada; [updated 2023 Mar 23]. Available from: https://www.canada.ca/en/radio-television-telecommunications/news/2023/03/crtc-to-improve-access-to-internet-and-mobile-services-across-canada.html

[15] Canada's Connectivity Strategy [Internet]. ISED Canada; [updated 2022 Apr 11]. Available from: https://ised-isde.canada.ca/site/high-speed-internet-canada/en/canadas-connectivity-strategy

[16] Connecting Families [Internet]. ISED Canada; [updated 2022 Oct 11]. Available from: https://ised-isde.canada.ca/site/connecting-families/en

The Role of Digital Health Policy and Leadership
K. Keshavjee and A. Khatami (Eds.)
© 2024 The Authors.
doi:10.3233/SHTI231323

Validation of a Design Architecture to Deliver Health Management and Behavior Change Evidence at Scale

Anson LI [a], Mark DAYOMI [b], Pooyeh GRAILI [b,c,d], Ali BALOUCHI [d], Aziz GUERGACHI [b,d,e] and Karim KESHAVJEE [b,1]

[a] *EY, Toronto, ON, Canada*
[b] *Institute for Health Policy, Management and Evaluation, Dalla Lana School of Public Health, University of Toronto, Toronto, ON, Canada*
[c] *Quality HTA, Oakville, ON, Canada*
[d] *Department of Information Technology Management, Ted Rogers School of Management, Toronto Metropolitan University, Toronto, ON, Canada*
[e] *Department of Mathematics and Statistics, York University, Toronto, ON, Canada*

Abstract. Forty-four percent of Canadians over the age of 20 have a non-communicable disease (NCD). Millions of Canadians are at risk of developing the complications of NCDs; millions have already experienced those complications. Fortunately, the evidence base for NCD prevention and behavior change is large and growing and digital technologies can deliver them at scale and with high fidelity. However, the current model of in-person primary care is not designed nor capable of operationalizing that evidence. New developments in artificial intelligence that can predict who will develop NCD or the complications of NCD are increasingly available, making the challenge of delivering disease prevention even more urgent. This paper presents findings from stakeholder engagement on a design architecture to address three initial barriers to large-scale deployment of health management and behavior change evidence: 1) the challenges of regulating mobile health apps, 2) the challenge of creating a value-based rationale for payers to invest in deploying mobile health apps at scale, and 3) the high cost of customer acquisition for delivering mobile health apps to those at risk.

Keywords. Disease prevention, mobile health apps, design architecture, platform, value-based care, behavior change, barriers

1. Introduction

The evidence base for disease and disease complication prevention is extremely large and growing rapidly. It is estimated that family physicians need to work 24 hours per day to provide all the care required by a typical 2000-patient practice. Primary care practices are designed for an investigate-assess-treat model of care but are poorly structured for the non-communicable disease (such as cardiovascular disease, diabetes, cancer, etc.) care model of educate-motivate-goal set-implement-monitor. The time needed for the latter model is significantly higher and requires a different approach.

---

[1] Corresponding Author: Karim Keshavjee karim.keshavjee@utoronto.ca

Mobile health applications (hApps) have demonstrated significant potential for improving patient care and health management and usage has increased over the last several years [1]. In the US, Kaiser Permanente developed a digital mental health and wellness ecosystem that includes health apps, patient-facing educational content, and workflow integration with electronic medical records [2]. The digital ecosystem increased patient engagement and improved daily function during treatment. In Germany, doctors can prescribe health apps that are reimbursed by the healthcare system, rather than paid for by the patient [3]. Several studies demonstrate the positive impact of hApps on health-related behaviors including physical activity, diet change, and adherence to medication or therapy [4]. Clinician adoption plays a critical role in the uptake and success of hApps [5,6]. The COVID-19 pandemic has increased end-user interest in hApps, however, hApps face several barriers to wider adoption. Barriers include unclear regulatory guidelines and policies, the high cost of customer acquisition, the lack of consumer willingness to pay [7], and poorly defined value propositions.

2. Methods

An environmental scan on patient accessibility to mobile health apps was conducted. A list of interest holders and their requirements for a hApp platform for patients was developed. Three key issues were identified that needed to be solved before other requirements could come into play. A first iteration of a proposed architecture was designed to solve those 3 key problems, described below. The proposed architecture was presented to a convenience sample of stakeholders (N=10) for validation. By architecture, we mean a minimal configuration of IT and non-IT components that deliver a specific desired functionality.

We asked interest holders their initial thoughts, what was attractive about the proposed architecture, what they were skeptical about, what they would do to improve it, whether it was feasible with their improvements, and suggestions to increase feasibility. The design architecture was iterated based on interest-holder feedback.

3. Proposed architecture to solve key problems in dissemination of health apps

3.1. Key issues that need to be addressed

Any marketplace for hApps cannot get off the ground if the following 3 key problems cannot be resolved:

- Is there a value proposition for at least one stakeholder to invest and overcome the lack of consumer willingness to pay?
- Can the value proposition be delivered at a cost and effort that is feasible?
- Can the marketplace be regulated and governed to deliver value and achieve sustainability?

3.2. Initial workflow to deliver the benefits

We developed a workflow that can deliver the benefits envisioned. The workflow is as follows: first, we identify disease areas with high economic burden, where effective treatments exist, AND where hApps are proven to make a difference. We then retrieve the current cost of treating the disease (usually in a hospital, but could also be in an outpatient setting) and then calculate the potential savings if existing evidence-based treatments could be delivered with higher fidelity to a larger number of affected individuals using hApps. We then calculate the value of cost-avoidance per patient and offer financial incentives that are attractive to hApp publishers to make their hApps available to patients with the disease, keeping costs lower than what can be saved; i.e., have a positive return on spending.

Second, we identify all the patients at the highest risk of getting the complication or exacerbation of the disease, which requires acute care, hospitalization or long-term outpatient treatment. This may require advanced predictive machine learning or artificial intelligence algorithms for early identification of an at-risk population. Many such algorithms already exist. Many more are under development. hApps are capable of monitoring the patient's health state if properly designed. Only patients at high risk of health system utilization are offered the hApp to maximize the cost-benefit ratio.

Lists of patients at high risk can be generated using the predictive algorithms in physician practices utilizing data that already exists in their EMRs. Physicians recommend a hApp from the Formulary list provided to them when the list of high-risk patients is generated. By involving physicians in the process, we identify the entire addressable market and decrease the cost of customer acquisition simultaneously. This maximizes the potential benefit of hApp dissemination and minimizes the costs. Physician compensation for their role in recommending and explaining the program to patients could be included in the Physician Schedule of Benefits.

Third, we propose a 'light' regulatory function that reviews the evidence for the use of the hApp, the usability evaluations and user experience reviews and that the hApp supports the latest guidelines for the disease in question. The hApp should be able to do 3 things to receive payment. First, it should be used by the user regularly. Second, it should collect data relevant to the disease or condition. Third, it should provide evidence-based advice to the patient. If the hApp meets all the requirements, it is given a conditional acceptance, which must be proven in actual usage; i.e., prevents the outcome of interest. The hApp is then listed on a formulary of approved products and communicated to physicians to recommend to identified, high-risk patients.

3.3. Draft design architecture

Figure 1 illustrates the draft design architecture for delivering the three minimum requirements needed to make large-scale hApp dissemination feasible. The data sources box allows for the training of machine learning and/or artificial intelligence algorithms that can identify at-risk patients at scale. The risk profiling service can help clinicians generate a list of high-risk patients in their EMR. The hApp Formulary service provides the physician with the list of approved hApps. The physician recommends the hApp to the patient using a QR code to minimize errors. The patient downloads it from the App Store after they scan the QR code.

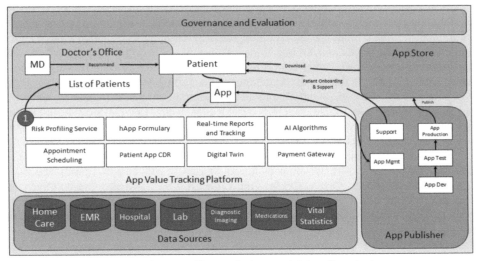

Figure 1. Reference architecture for large-scale hApp dissemination.

In this model, App Publishers are incentivized to ensure patients are properly onboarded and supported since payments depend on patients having a successful experience with the hApp. The Governance and Evaluation function provides regulatory oversight and ensures that value for money is being delivered. hApps that don't deliver value are deprecated from the Formulary if they do not meet pre-set criteria after a reasonable period; e.g., an 18-24 probationary period.

3.4. Example of potential use case

The economic burden of end-stage renal disease (ESRD) in Canada is high, estimated at more than $4.5 billion per year in Canada [8]. Dialysis treatment for patients with ESRD is one of the most expensive medical treatments, costing over $1.8 billion per year in Canada. Currently, the most significant contributors of ESRD in patients are diabetes (38.0%) and hypertension (12.2%).

Patients at risk of developing ESRD, their family physicians, and the Canadian healthcare system could benefit from the model proposed in Sections 3.2 and 3.3. At-risk patients can be identified from data in EMRs through the App Value Tracking Platform. Family physicians can prescribe relevant health apps from the formulary list, such as hApps that track and remind patients to take their blood pressure medications. This can help reduce the risk of patients developing ESRD, thus reducing the financial burden of ESRD on the Canadian healthcare system.

4.   Stakeholder feedback on the design architecture

First impressions. The concept received positive overall feedback and optimism and garnered interest from the interviewed stakeholders. This positivity was balanced with pragmatic considerations for operationalizing the platform effectively and ethically.

Features –attractive. Interviewees widely appreciated the concept of a hApp marketplace. Several praised the ability of hApps to extend healthcare services beyond traditional facilities, reducing the strain on practitioners and the system at large. Others valued the model for its aim to engage payers, promote preventative care, and use AI and advanced analytics to identify and manage at-risk patients. Similarly, the technical architecture, which facilitates the matching of the right hAapps to the right patients, was acknowledged for its potential to reduce waste, improve health outcomes, and curb costs. One interviewee also favored the idea of using the platform as a digital pharmacy, where practitioners could digitally prescribe apps to patients, akin to prescribing medications.

Features –skeptical. Interviewees expressed scepticism over several element of the platform. Some were uneasy about using AI to find at-risk patients, citing the poor quality of medical data, particularly for vulnerable groups. A patient representative was particularly doubtful about whether different groups like the elderly and immigrants would adopt the solution and stressed the need for educating potential users and medical professionals. Some participants questioned the proposed financial plan, technical setup, and the platform's security measures. Concerns extended to market forces such as the competitive hApp landscape and the challenges of integrating existing apps.

Areas for improvement. There were many suggestions to make the hApp platform better, including advice for successful implementation, compatibility with multiple hApps, and ease of use. Interviewees mentioned the importance of keeping user data safe, having a clear business model, and making sure doctors and other stakeholders are on board with the idea. They also stressed making the platform accessible to everyone, including older people, and ensuring that the hApps on the platform were effective and trustworthy. Lastly, interviewees called for better hApp vetting protocols and governance on the platform to maximize clinical benefits.

Assessment of feasibility. There were varying views on the platform's feasibility. Some saw the proposal as promising but suggested a cautious, phased rollout. Others emphasized the need for careful design and experimentation. Others pointed out potential hurdles like getting physician buy-in, challenges with value-based payments, and the readiness of primary care teams for a surge of apps. A few interviewees highlighted the importance of making the platform appealing to both doctors and patients. Some were cautiously optimistic, acknowledging the implementation complexities but appreciating the potential benefits. They suggested refining the approach to match patients with relevant apps better. Overall, most interviewees thought the concept was technically and conceptually feasible, as long as key implementation issues were addressed.

Improving feasibility. Many interviewees advocated for a staged deployment of the platform, initiating particular diseases, and fostering trust with users by offering valuable services. They propose establishing a robust technical framework with an open design that can accommodate various hApps, complemented by a user-friendly interface. Certain experts stressed the importance of validating the hApp's effectiveness through trials and ongoing feedback. They also recommended forming close collaborations with healthcare organizations and governmental bodies for support, coupled with clear guidelines for hApp assessment. Promoting innovation and tackling privacy issues was deemed crucial, alongside redirecting focus to demonstrate how the platform can positively impact employment and the economy. Another common suggestion was the need for government support and new payment models to ensure the success of the platform. Overall, we collected a list of over a dozen 'known issues' that need to be answered to make the project acceptable to a wider audience.

5. Discussion and Conclusion

This study adds to the literature on methods to make hApps available to patients at scale. Interest holders identified many issues that must be overcome to make a hApp platform a reality. Two key areas that need to be addressed include patient education about AI and its value in helping them achieve their health goals and creating a compelling business case for funders to invest in a hApp platform.

Limitations of the study include the small sample size and the limited number of interest holders engaged. Through the interest-holder interviews, we identified over a dozen requirements that need to be addressed to make the platform potentially attractive to additional interest holders. Future research needs to focus on making the platform attractive to physicians, as their role is critical to the success of such a platform. Future interest holder engagement will also address patient concerns and hesitations, the role of researchers, the implementation details for hApp-related payments, and who should provide the governance and evaluation function.

Successful deployment of the hApp platform will require overcoming operational, ethical, and inclusivity challenges. Enabling the direct transfer of evidence-based knowledge to patients, the hApp platform holds the potential to revolutionize patient education and monitoring, particularly for those at risk of non-communicable diseases. This advancement could mark a significant shift towards a more proactive and patient-centered healthcare system.

References

[1]   Kao CK, Liebovitz DM. Consumer Mobile Health Apps: Current State, Barriers, and Future Directions. PM R. 2017 May;9(5S):S106-S115. doi: 10.1016/j.pmrj.2017.02.018. PMID: 28527495.
[2]   Mordecai D, Histon T, Neuwirth E, Heisler S., et al. How Kaiser Permanente Created a Mental Health and Wellness Digital Ecosystem [Internet]. New England Journal of Medicine; 2021 [cited 2023 Dec 17]. Available from: https://catalyst.nejm.org/doi/full/10.1056/CAT.20.0295
[3]   Digital Health Applications (DiGA) [Internet]. Federal Institute for Drugs and Medical Devices; 2019 [cited 2023 Dec 17]. Available from: https://www.bfarm.de/EN/Medical-devices/Tasks/DiGA-and-DiPA/Digital-Health-Applications/_node. html
[4]   Han M, Lee E. Effectiveness of Mobile Health Application Use to Improve Health Behavior Changes: A Systematic Review of Randomized Controlled Trials. Healthc Inform Res. 2018 Jul;24(3):207-226. doi: 10.4258/hir.2018.24.3.207. Epub 2018 Jul 31. PMID: 30109154; PMCID: PMC6085201.
[5]   Jacob C, Sanchez-Vazquez A, Ivory C. Understanding Clinicians' Adoption of Mobile Health Tools: A Qualitative Review of the Most Used Frameworks. JMIR Mhealth Uhealth 2020;8(7):e18072
[6]   Chindalo P, Karim A, Brahmbhatt R, Saha N, Keshavjee K. Health apps by design: a reference architecture for mobile engagement. In Health Care Delivery and Clinical Science: Concepts, Methodologies, Tools, and Applications 2018 (pp. 553-563). IGI Global.
[7]   Deal K, Keshavjee K, Troyan S, Kyba R, Holbrook AM. Physician and patient willingness to pay for electronic cardiovascular disease management. Int J Med Inform. 2014 Jul;83(7):517-28. doi: 10.1016/j.ijmedinf.2014.04.007. Epub 2014 Apr 29. PMID: 24862891.
[8]   Kitzler TM, Chun J. Understanding the Current Landscape of Kidney Disease in Canada to Advance Precision Medicine Guided Personalized Care. Can J Kidney Health Dis. 2023 Feb 13;10:20543581231154185. doi: 10.1177/20543581231154185. PMID: 36798634; PMCID: PMC9926383.

Subject Index

The Role of Digital Health Policy and Leadership
K. Keshavjee and A. Khatami (Eds.)
© 2024 The Authors.
This article is published online with Open Access by IOS Press and distributed under the terms
of the Creative Commons Attribution Non-Commercial License 4.0 (CC BY-NC 4.0).

Author Index